Geriatric Fracture: Current Treatment and Future Options

Geriatric Fracture: Current Treatment and Future Options

Guest Editors

Detlef Van der Velde
Henk Jan Schuijt

MDPI Basel • Beijing • Wuhan • Barcelona • Belgrade • Novi Sad • Cluj • Manchester

Guest Editors

Detlef Van der Velde
Department of Geriatric Trauma
St. Antonius Hospital
Utrecht
The Netherlands

Henk Jan Schuijt
Department of Geriatric Trauma
St. Antonius Hospital
Utrecht
The Netherlands

Editorial Office
MDPI AG
Grosspeteranlage 5
4052 Basel, Switzerland

This is a reprint of the Special Issue, published open access by the journal *Journal of Clinical Medicine* (ISSN 2077-0383), freely accessible at: https://www.mdpi.com/journal/jcm/special_issues/CK93S5G970.

For citation purposes, cite each article independently as indicated on the article page online and as indicated below:

Lastname, A.A.; Lastname, B.B. Article Title. *Journal Name* **Year**, *Volume Number*, Page Range.

ISBN 978-3-7258-5451-6 (Hbk)
ISBN 978-3-7258-5452-3 (PDF)
https://doi.org/10.3390/books978-3-7258-5452-3

Contents

About the Editors

Detlef van der Velde

Detlef van der Velde is a trauma surgeon and principal investigator at St. Antonius Hospital in Nieuwegein, Netherlands, specializing in geriatric trauma care. He is a pioneer who established the first geriatric trauma unit in the Netherlands, focusing on optimizing outcomes for older adults with traumatic injuries. His research interests include hip fractures, shared decision-making in geriatric trauma, and the integration of palliative care in trauma management. He has authored numerous publications in these areas; in addition to his clinical and research roles, Dr. van der Velde is an advocate for improving the quality of care for older trauma patients and has been involved in various initiatives to enhance multidisciplinary collaboration in geriatric trauma care.

Henk Jan Schuijt

Henk Jan Schuijt is a resident and postdoctoral researcher in geriatric medicine, with a special interest in geriatric trauma care, at Amsterdam University Medical Centre and Center for Geriatric Trauma at Antonius Hospital, NL. He completed his PhD at Utrecht University in 2021, focusing on cultural change in geriatric traumatology, and now combines clinical practice with research aimed at improving outcomes for older adults with traumatic injuries.

He is actively involved in multiple national consortia, implementation studies, and contributes to the Netherlands Implementation Collective, applying implementation science to enhance research impact and clinical care.

Journal of
Clinical Medicine

MDPI

Systematic Review

Reverse Shoulder Arthroplasty versus Non-Operative Treatment of Three-Part and Four-Part Proximal Humerus Fractures in the Elderly Patient: A Pooled Analysis and Systematic Review

Thomas P. Bosch [1,2,*], Frank J. P. Beeres [1,3], Steven Ferree [4], Inger B. Schipper [2], Roland S. Camenzind [3], Ruben J. Hoepelman [4], Björn-Christian Link [3], Ingmar F. Rompen [5], Reto Babst [1,3] and Bryan J. M. van de Wall [1,3]

1 Department of Health Sciences and Medicine, University of Lucerne, 6002 Luzern, Switzerland
2 Department of Trauma Surgery, Leiden University Medical Centre, 2300 RC Leiden, The Netherlands
3 Department of Orthopedics and Trauma Surgery, Lucerne Cantonal Hospital, 6000 Luzern, Switzerland
4 Department of Surgery, University Medical Center Utrecht, 3584 CX Utrecht, The Netherlands; r.j.hoepelman-2@umcutrecht.nl (R.J.H.)
5 Department of Surgery, University Hospital Heidelberg, 69117 Heidelberg, Germany
* Correspondence: t.p.bosch@lumc.nl

Abstract: Background: The treatment of complex proximal humerus fractures in elderly patients is not yet fully elucidated. Of all treatment options, reverse shoulder arthroplasty (RSA) and non-operative treatment (NOT) appear to provide the best results. Evidence to guide the choice between the two is sparse. Therefore, this review provides an overview of the available evidence on RSA versus NOT. **Methods**: Studies comparing complex proximal humerus fractures in patients aged >65 years treated either with RSA or NOT were included for systematic review and direct comparison via pooled analysis of patient-rated outcome and range of motion. Indirect comparison of case series and non-comparative studies on either treatment was performed separately. **Results**: Three comparative studies including 77 patients treated with RSA and 81 treated non-operatively were analysed. The RSA group scored better for both the Constant–Murley score (mean difference 6 points) and DASH score (mean difference 8 points). No differences were detected in ASES, PENN score, pain scores, or range of motion between treatment groups. The most common complications for RSA were infection (3%), nerve injury (2%), and dislocation (2%). Reoperation was required in 5%. In the NOT group, common complications included malunion (42%), osteonecrosis (25%), and non-union (3%); no reoperation was required. Patient satisfaction was equal in both groups. **Conclusions**: The functional outcomes and range of motion after RSA seemed satisfactory and potentially superior to NOT in elderly patients. Patient satisfaction was comparable despite a high malunion and osteonecrosis rate in the non-operative treatment group, which did not require re-interventions.

Keywords: arthroplasty complications; complex humerus fracture; frail trauma patient; non-operative treatment; reverse shoulder arthroplasty

1. Introduction

Proximal humerus fractures (PHFs) are common injuries and account for 5% of all adult fractures [1]. They represent one of the most common fractures in elderly patients with poor bone quality. Due to an aging population, their incidence is expected to rise in the upcoming decades, increasing costs and burden on an already stretched healthcare system. Optimising the treatment of these fractures is vital to keeping our healthcare system sustainable.

Treatment options in elderly patients with PHF generally consist of non-operative treatment (NOT), open reduction and internal fixation (ORIF), hemiarthroplasty (HA), and reverse total shoulder arthroplasty (RSA). Frequently, the Neer classification is used to guide treatment decisions. The Neer classification categorises PHFs based on the number and displacement of fracture fragments [2]. Simple PHFs are generally treated non-operatively with satisfactory results. With increasing complexity of the fracture pattern, outcomes are thought to be poorer when left untouched. As a result, surgeons frequently revert to one of the aforementioned surgical treatment options to counteract this inverse relation. The advantage of ORIF is that the native joint is preserved, generally offering better functional results than arthroplasty. However, elderly patients are at a considerable risk of developing humeral head necrosis, potentially necessitating arthroplasty when symptomatic. Offering primary arthroplasty for fractures has the benefit of preventing secondary surgery related to failure of ORIF. However, when complications such as infection occur, they may have disastrous consequences for patients [3].

The debate on the optimal treatment modality in elderly patients with three- or four-part PHF is still ongoing. Several randomized studies and meta-analysis found no added benefit of surgical management with ORIF or HA compared to NOT [4,5]. However, studies did find better outcomes for patients treated with RSA compared with ORIF or HA [6–8].

RSA has become an increasingly popular surgical modality for treating three- and four-part proximal humerus fractures [9]. Its superior results in comparison to other surgical options in recent studies could be an explanation for its growing use. However, in elderly patients, range of motion and functional outcome after NOT appear to be acceptable as well, even in displaced fractures [4,5,10,11]. To date, there have been no systematic reviews comparing the results of NOT with those of RSA for treatment of three- and four-part proximal humerus fractures.

The goal of this systematic review is to compare the patient-reported functional outcome and range of motion of RSA compared with NOT in elderly patients who sustained three- or four-part proximal humerus fractures.

2. Methods

This study was set up as a systematic review to be performed according to the Preferred Reporting Items for Systematic Reviews and Meta-analysis (PRISMA) checklist [12] and Meta-analysis of Observational Studies in Epidemiology (MOOSE) [13]. No protocol has been published for this study.

2.1. Search Strategy and Selection Criteria

Databases of PubMed, Embase, CINAHL, and CENTRAL were searched on 18 January 2023 for studies on complex proximal humerus fractures in patients aged 65 years and older comparing RSA to NOT (Supplementary Material Table S1). Two reviewers screened titles and abstracts independently for eligibility. All studies comparing RSA and NOT were included for systematic review and (if possible) direct comparison via pooled analysis. Indirect comparison via systematic review of case series and non-comparative studies on either of the two treatment modalities was performed separately.

Full-text screening was performed by the same authors. Inclusion criteria were comparative studies on RSA versus NOT for treatment of complex proximal humeral fractures (classified as Neer three- or four-part displaced or AO (Arbeitsgemeinschaft für Osteosynthesefragen) classification 11-B or 11-C), age over 65 years (when not specified in the inclusion criteria, then mean age of 70 or older in the baseline characteristics), functional outcome and/or range of motion reported with a minimal follow up of 12 months. Non-operative treatment was defined as no invasive intervention performed (thus excluding open and closed reduction with or without Kirschner wire fixation). Exclusion criteria were congress or meeting abstracts, biomechanical, animal, or cadaver studies, no English, Dutch, or German full text available. Disagreements on study eligibility and quality were discussed and the decision to perform meta-analysis was reached through consensus of the authors. Reviews of the references of included studies were performed to identify studies missed in the initial search.

2.2. Data Extraction

One author extracted the data using a prespecified extraction sheet, includingyear of publication, study design, time period of study, follow up, patient characteristics, fracture classification and distribution, prosthesis type, cemented yes/no, approach used, reinsertion of tuberosities yes/no, outcome scores, pain score, and satisfaction with treatment modality. Regarding complications, the following were extracted from the studies: radiographic outcomes including loosening of stem or baseplate, scapular notching, and anatomic tuberosity healing for the RSA group and nonunion, malunion, and osteonecrosis for the NOT group. Furthermore, infection, dislocation, iatrogenic fracture, and revision surgery were noted.

2.3. Quality Assessment

The included studies were assessed by one author using the Methodological Index for Non-Randomized Studies (MINORS) tool. This validated tool for assessing methodological quality of studies rates studies from scores 0 to 24 (Supplementary Material Table S2). Pooled analysis was performed only when the following criteria were met: equivalence of baseline characteristics in the two treatment groups and availability of a minimum of three studies reporting on the outcome(s) of interest.

2.4. Study Outcome

The primary outcomes were functional outcome scores and range of motion after at least 12 months. Secondary outcomes were all complications, pain, and satisfaction with treatment.

2.5. Statistical Analysis

Variables were presented as per the original studies. Weighted average and mean difference of outcome scores were calculated when more than two studies reported on the same scale or questionnaire. The pooled mean scores were calculated through weighting of study size. Excel was used for data collection, calculation of pooling results, and analysis.

3. Results

The flowchart of the literature search and comparative study selection is shown in Figure 1. Three studies were included; one randomized clinical trial (Lopiz et al.) and two retrospective cohort studies (Chivot et al. and Roberson et al.) [14–16].

3.1. Comparative Studies

3.1.1. Study Characteristics and Quality Assessment

The three studies included 158 patients; 77 underwent RSA and 81 had NOT. Table 1 provides the baseline characteristics of the studies. Lopiz et al. [14] and Roberson et al. [16] both included more (87% and 75% respectively) four-part fractures than Chivot et al. [15] Roberson et al. [16] included patients in the NOT group who were offered RSA as indicated by the surgeon but declined. The percentage lost to follow-up was 5% in the study by Lopiz et al. [14], 50% for Chivot et al. [15], and Roberson et al. did not provide data on eligible numbers of patients or follow-up. Table 2 shows the MINORS scores ranging from 13 to 24. In all included studies, the deltopectoral approach was used for the placement of the RSA.

3.1.2. Functional Outcomes

Two studies [14,15] reported on the Constant–Murley score (CMS). The scores appeared to be significantly better in the RSA group in both studies, with a mean difference of six points (Table 3). Two studies [14,15] reported on the Disability of the Arm, Shoulder and Hand Questionnaire (DASH) score. The randomized clinical trial found a significantly better score in the RSA group, with a difference of eight points. One observational study found approximately the same difference in favour of RSA, but this was not statistically significant. No differences were found in the American Shoulder and Elbow Surgeons shoulder score (ASES) or Penn shoulder score (PENN) in the two studies that reported on these outcomes.

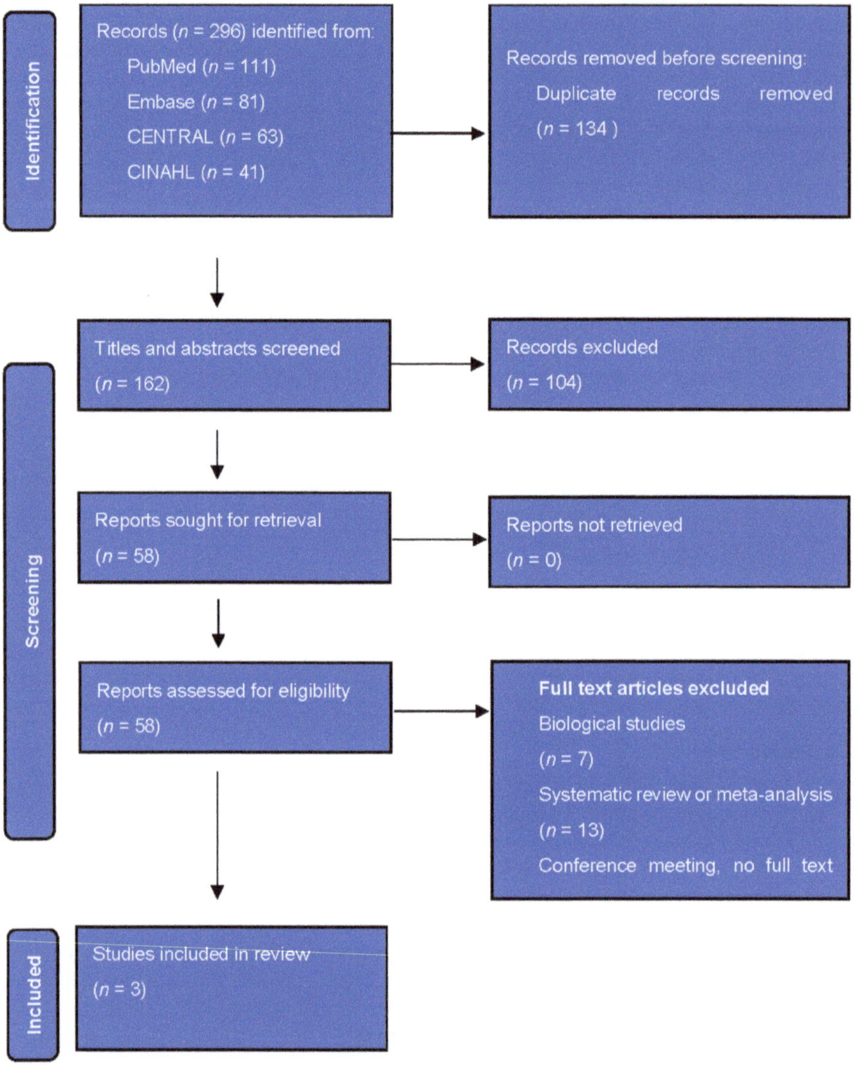

Figure 1. Flow diagram of search and selection of comparative studies.

3.1.3. Range of Motion

Chivot et al. [15] found better ROM in the RSA group for all movements. Lopiz et al. [14] found better anterior elevation in the RSA group compared with NOT but not better external or internal rotation. Abduction was investigated only by Lopiz et al. [14] and they found no difference (abduction >90 degree; RSA 72% versus NOT 42%, p0.064). Roberson found no improvements in anterior elevation or external rotation (Table 4).

Table 1. Baseline characteristics of studies after reverse total shoulder arthroplasty versus non-operative treatment.

Author	Design	Number of Patients		Age Mean in Years (Sd)		% Female		% Neer 4-part		Tuberculum Management	Prothesis Used	Follow-Up Months
		RSA	NOT	RSA	NOT	RSA	NOT	RSA	NOT			Average
Lopiz	RCT	29	30	82 (3.4)	85 (4.8)	86%	87%	87%	83%	Reattachment	Delta SMR	12
Chivot	Retro	28	32	77 (70–92)	79 (70–92)	78.6%	93.8%	35.7%	25%	Reattachment	Zimmer	32
Roberson	Retro	20	19	71 (NR)	71 (NR)	95%	78.9%	75%	21%	NR	DJO Zimmer	29/53 ^
		77	81									

Retro: retrospective study, RCT: randomized clinical trial, RSA: reversed total shoulder arthroplasty, NOT: non-operative treatment, NR: not reported, Delta: Delta XTEND Reverse Shoulder System prosthesis (DePuy, Warsaw, IN, USA), SMR: SMR Modular Shoulder System (Systema Multiplana Randelli; Lima-LTO, San Daniele del Friuli, Italy), Zimmer: The Trabecular Metal Reverse Shoulder System implant (Zimmer Biomet, Warsaw, IN, USA), DJO: Reverse Shoulder Prosthesis (DJO Surgical, Austin, TX, USA), ^: follow-up NOT group 29 months, RSA group 53 months.

Table 2. Quality assessment for studies after reverse total shoulder arthroplasty versus non-operative treatment.

	Randomized Clinical Trials	Lopiz 2019 [14]	Retrospective Studies	Chivot 2018 [15]	Roberson 2017 [16]
Clearly stated aim		2		2	2
Inclusion of consecutive patients		2		2	1
Prospective data collection		2		1	0
Appropriate endpoints		2		2	1
Unbiased assessment endpoints		2		0	0
Appropriate follow-up (>1 year)		2		2	2
Loss to follow-up <5%		2		1	0
Prospective calculation study size		2		0	0
Adequate control group		2		2	2
Contemporary groups		2		2	2
Baseline quivalence of groups		2		2	2
Adequate statistical analysis		2		2	1
Total score		24		18	13

3.1.4. Complications

An overview of the complications for both RSA and NOT in the three included comparative studies is given in Table 5. In total there were four (5%) reoperations reported in the three studies; two for infection (one debridement and implant retention procedure and one removal of prosthesis), one for dislocation of the RSA, and one for postoperative stiffness.

3.1.5. Pain and Satisfaction

Only Lopiz et al. [14] reported less pain in the RSA group, with VAS 0.9 versus 1.6 in the NOT group (p = 0.011). Roberson and Chivot et al. found no differences in pain scores [15,16].

With regard to treatment satisfaction, Lopiz et al. [14] reported that 100% of the RSA group versus 93% in NOT 'would undergo the same treatment again based on the achieved result' ($p = 0.24$). Chivot et al. also found higher satisfaction in the RSA group, with 93% versus 84% in the NOT group ($p = 0.03$).

Table 3. Functional outcome scores after reverse total shoulder arthroplasty versus non-operative treatment.

Functional Outcome Score	Study	RSA	NOT	p-Value
CMS *	Lopiz et al. [14]	61.7	55.7	0.07
	Chivot et al. [15]	56.5	50.5	**0.03** ^
DASH **	Lopiz et al. [14]	20.7	28.8	0.08
	Chivot et al. [15]	38.7	31.2	0.11
PENN *	Roberson et al. [16]	70	73	0.7
ASES *	Roberson et al. [16]	72	72	0.99

CMS: Constant–Murley Score, DASH: Disability of the Arm, Shoulder and Hand questionnaire, ASES: American Shoulder and Elbow Surgeons shoulder score, PENN: Penn shoulder score, RSA: reverse shoulder arthroplasty, NOT: non-operative treatment, *: ranging 0–100 with higher score indicating better function, **: ranging 0–100 with lower score indicating better function, ^: difference in favour of RSA.

Table 4. Range-of-motion scores after reverse total shoulder arthroplasty versus non-operative treatment.

Range of Motion	Study	RSA	NOT	p-Value
Forward flexion	Lopiz et al. [14]	133	115	**0.028** ^
	Chivot et al. [15]	110	98	**0.0005** ^
	Roberson et al. [16]	119	120	0.87
	Weighted average	120.8	109.8	
External rotation	Lopiz et al. * [14]	5.2	4.4	0.293
	Chivot et al. [15]	19	9	**0.0002** ^
	Roberson et al. [16]	31	23	0.06
Internal rotation **	Lopiz et al. [14]	65% (41/24)	48% (34/14)	0.211
	Chivot et al. [15]	46% (17/28)	22% (9/13)	**0.04** ^

RSA: reverse shoulder arthroplasty, NOT: non-operative treatment, *: range of motion part of Constant–Murley Score, **: percentage patients with internal rotation above sacro-iliac joint level, (% lumbar/% thoracic), ^: difference in favour of RSA.

Table 5. Complications in included studies after RSA and NOT for proximal humerus fracture in elderly patients.

	RSA	NOT
N	77	81
RSA complications		
Dislocation	2 (2.6%)	
Nerve injury	2 (2.6%)	
Infection	2 (2.6%)	
Iatrogenic fracture	0	
Anatomic greater tuberosity healing	40 (52%)	
Greater tuberosity non-anatomic healing or resorption	17 (22%)	
Scapular notching	0	
Baseplate loosening	0	
Humeral stem loosening	0	
Revision or subsequent operation	4 (5.2%)	0
NOT complications		
Osteonecrosis		20 (24.7%)
Malunion		34 (42%)
Nonunion		2 (2.5%)

N: number, RSA: reverse shoulder arthroplasty, NOT: non-operative treatment.

3.1.6. Case Series and Non-Comparative Studies on RSA and NOT

A total of 29 studies (1550 patients) reporting on RSA in case series or comparing elderly patients treated for complex proximal humeral fractures with treatments other than NOT were included for review of functionality and range-of-motion outcomes and complications [7,8,17–43]. Five case series and non-comparative studies after NOT were included (249 patients) (Supplementary Materials Tables S4 and S6) [10,44–47]. Weighted mean functional outcome scores after RSA were CMS 60, DASH 25, ASES 76, OSS 39, and Simple Shoulder Test 7.8 (Supplementary Materials Table S5). For NOT, the weighted mean scores were CMS 60, DASH 33.0, and OSS 36 (Supplementary Materials Table S6). Range of motion in degrees after RSA was anterior elevation 122, abduction 112, and external rotation 22 (Supplementary Materials Table S5). Twenty-five studies reported complications after RSA. The average rate of complications was 4.6% (infection 2%, dislocation 1.6%, and iatrogenic fracture 1%). The revision rate for infection, dislocation, iatrogenic fracture, or aseptic loosening in all studies averaged 4%.

4. Discussion

This review describes the differences in functional outcomes after RSA versus NOT in elderly patients with complex proximal humerus fractures. Functional outcomes and range of motion after RSA seemed better compared with NOT in comparative studies. The rate of complications after RSA was low at 3%, with an overall revision rate of 5%.

So, what are the clinical implications following these findings? It is likely that surgeons will have treated-higher demand patients with more complex fractures with RSA and lower-demand, less complex fractures non-operatively. This assumption is based on the fact that multiple case series have mentioned this in relation to their patient selection for RSA [7,8,20,23,33]. Although only discussed in one of the included observational comparative studies, it is likely that this was also the case here [16]. The big question remains: to what extent are the better results found in the RSA group attributable to the treatment itself and not to the type of patient (high-demand) or the complexity of the fracture? The one RCT included in this review that could have shed some light on this matter did not find any statistical significant difference in functional outcomes; however, scores for all outcomes were consistently better in the RSA group. On top of that, the large quantity of non-comparative studies point in the same direction, so it may be safe to say that RSA is likely to have some beneficial effect on patient outcomes. The magnitude of this effect remains unclear and should be further investigated.

Nevertheless, the results of this review still are valuable; they contribute to the knowledge on specific aspects of this topic. Assuming a selection bias to be present, the results shows that if we continue to offer RSA to high-demand patients with complex fractures and non-operative treatment to the lower-demand patients with less complex fractures, we can achieve satisfactory results in our day-to-day practice. It would be interesting to see future studies taking this confounding factor out of the equation, to truly understand how both treatment modalities behave in both the high-demand/complex fracture and low-demand/low complex fracture patient population.

A pragmatic approach in the treatment of elderly patients with complex proximal humerus fractures could be to consider RSA in cases where NOT has led to unfavourable outcomes. Several studies have shown that delayed RSA (>30 days) provides equal functional outcomes and range of motion to early RSA (<30 days) [16,48–50]. Interestingly, patients treated with RSA for sequalae of NOT potentially outperform patients after NOT on both functionality and range-of-motion scores [51]. In other words, conservative management and offering RSA either directly or in cases of failed conservative treatment, are both viable strategies for treating complex proximal humerus fractures in the elderly.

Non-anatomic healing and resorption of the greater tuberosity is frequently seen in patients who undergo RSA. The clinical relevance of this occurrence remains questionable. Several studies found that it was related to poor functional outcomes and range of motion. However, an equal number of studies did not find such a relation [24]. Therefore, it remains unclear whether non-anatomic healing and resorption should be regarded as complications or not. The same applies for malunion and osteonecrosis in the NOT group. These are regarded as complications; however, their relevance is questionable. Many patients with osteonecrosis are asymptomatic and do not require intervention [52]. Moreover, malunion is practically assured when complex fractures are treated conservatively. This is also reflected in the results of the present study; despite the high incidence of malunion and osteonecrosis, reintervention rates were low in the NOT group. It should, however, be acknowledged that it remains unclear whether a deliberate choice to refrain from revision surgery was made (for example because of severe comorbidities) or patients were truly satisfied with the results.

With regard to risk of other complications (infection, dislocation, nerve injury, reintervention) with RSA, it should be kept in mind that although complication and revision rates are low and long-term follow-up of RSA shows high arthroplasty survival rates and good clinical results, these results deteriorate over time [53]. Complication rates also appear to increase over time [54]. Furthermore, as previously stated, revision rate is not the same as success rate. An elderly patient with complications after initial RSA might not consent to revision surgery and might accept a less favourable result than would have been achieved with NOT. It is thus unclear whether the advantage of RSA over NOT is sustained over time and whether it is worth the risk of complications.

The burden on the healthcare system due to fractures has grown exponentially in recent decades. This is mainly attributed to a continuously expanding and aging population with higher expectations in the context of an increasingly demanding society [1,55]. Inevitably, the increased burden poses higher costs, putting the sustainability of countries' healthcare systems at risk [56,57]. As PHFs are the second most common fractures in elderly people after hip fractures, it is important to consider the costs associated with the treatment of complex PHFs. The initial costs of RSA are higher than NOT, as expected, because of the cost associated with facilitating an RSA operation and the duration of the hospital stay. Yet, these costs seem to pay out over time. In 2022, Abdel Khalik et al. conducted a cost–utility analysis comparing HA, ORIF, RSA, and NOT in elderly patients, aged 75 years and older, with complex proximal humerus fractures. The study determined the reported inpatient cost QALY ratio in NOT and RSA to be 2584 CAD/QALY and 3077 CAD/QALY, respectively. Despite these higher upfront costs, RSA was deemed a more cost-effective treatment strategy for complex proximal humerus fractures in patients older than 65 years compared with NOT, because of its superiority in functional and clinical outcomes over time even in the older population [58].

5. Limitations

This review highlights the advantages of RSA compared with NOT. To our knowledge, this is the first review to address outcomes after RSA versus NOT for complex proximal humerus fractures specifically in elderly patients. Unfortunately, no meta-analysis was possible due to the small number of studies comparing only three-part and four-part proximal humerus fractures and heterogeneity in the study population (age and fracture type). Another limitation of our review is the lack of non-comparative studies reporting on NOT outcomes to put the results in perspective, like the extensive data on RSA outcomes. Finally, as previously stated, it is likely that selection bias might have occurred in the included observational studies and case series.

6. Conclusions

The functional outcomes and range of motion after RSA seem satisfactory and potentially superior to those achieved with NOT in elderly patients. The complication rate was acceptably low and an overall revision rate of 5% was found. These results should, however, be viewed in light of distinct differences in patient characteristics between treatment groups.

Which geriatric patients with complex proximal humerus fractures benefit from RSA should be the focus of future research. The NITEP (https://pubmed.ncbi.nlm.nih.gov/30700485/, accessed on 16 April 2024) and ReShAPE trials (https://pubmed.ncbi.nlm.nih.gov/30700485/, accessed on 16 April 2024) might shed some light on this topic and guide future treatment choices.

7. Future Directions

To further explore which elderly PHF patients most benefit from NOT and which from RSA without potential selection bias, a randomized controlled trial comparing treatment modalities including an adequate sample size and follow-up time is necessary. Furthermore, future studies should incorporate comprehensive assessments of both clinical and radiographic outcomes, including functional recovery, pain relief, range of motion, fracture healing, and implant positioning. Follow-up should extend beyond one year to evaluate the durability of treatment effects and the occurrence of late complications. Additionally, subgroup analyses based on patient characteristics and fracture patterns should be conducted to identify factors predictive of treatment success and guide physicians in personalised treatment decisions. Ultimately, the findings from future studies will contribute to facilitating evidence-based guidelines and improving the management of complex proximal humerus fractures in the elderly, enhancing patient outcomes and quality of life.

Supplementary Materials: The following supporting information can be downloaded at https://www.mdpi.com/article/10.3390/jcm13113344/s1: Table S1: Syntax of literature search on reverse total shoulder arthroplasty compared with non-operative treatment for proximal humeral fractures in the elderly; Table S2: Quality assessment according to the MINORS criteria; Table S3: Baseline characteristics of non-comparative studies and case series on RSA; Table S4: Functional outcome scores and weighted mean scores of case series and non-comparative studies on RSA; Table S5: Range of motion and weighted mean scores of case series and non-comparative studies on RSA; Table S6: Functional outcome scores and weighted mean scores of NOT cohorts from studies not compared with RSA.

Author Contributions: Conceptualization was conducted by B.J.M.v.d.W., R.B. and F.J.P.B., T.P.B. and S.F. carried out the literature search and extracted data. R.S.C. and R.J.H. caried out further investigation and data curation. B.-C.L. and I.F.R. managed resources and project administration. Disagreements on study eligibility and quality were discussed and the decision to perform meta-analysis was reached through consensus of the authors: S.F., T.P.B. and F.J.P.B. Supervision was carried out by B.J.M.v.d.W. and I.B.S. All authors have read and agreed to the published version of the manuscript.

Funding: This research received no external funding.

Conflicts of Interest: The authors declare no conflicts of interest.

References

1. Court-Brown, C.M.; Caesar, B. Epidemiology of Adult Fractures: A Review. *Injury* **2006**, *37*, 691–697. [CrossRef]
2. Carofino, B.C.; Leopold, S.S. Classifications in Brief: The Neer Classification for Proximal Humerus Fractures. *Clin. Orthop. Relat. Res.* **2013**, *471*, 39–43. [CrossRef]
3. Grammont, P.; Trouilloud, P.; Laffay, J.; Deries, X. Study and Development of a New Shoulder Prosthesis. *Rhumatologie* **1987**, *39*, 407–418.
4. Olerud, P.; Ahrengart, L.; Ponzer, S.; Saving, J.; Tidermark, J. Hemiarthroplasty Versus Nonoperative Treatment of Displaced 4-Part Proximal Humeral Fractures in Elderly Patients: A Randomized Controlled Trial. *J. Shoulder Elb. Surg.* **2011**, *20*, 1025–1033. [CrossRef]
5. Olerud, P.; Ahrengart, L.; Ponzer, S.; Saving, J.; Tidermark, J. Internal Fixation Versus Nonoperative Treatment of Displaced 3-Part Proximal Humeral Fractures in Elderly Patients: A Randomized Controlled Trial. *J. Shoulder Elb. Surg.* **2011**, *20*, 747–755. [CrossRef]
6. Orman, S.; Mohamadi, A.; Serino, J.; Murphy, J.; Hanna, P.; Weaver, M.J.; Dyer, G.; Nazarian, A.; von Keudell, A. Comparison of Surgical and Non-Surgical Treatments for 3- and 4-Part Proximal Humerus Fractures: A Network Meta-Analysis. *Shoulder Elb.* **2020**, *12*, 99–108. [CrossRef]
7. Cuff, D.J.; Pupello, D.R. Comparison of Hemiarthroplasty and Reverse Shoulder Arthroplasty for the Treatment of Proximal Humeral Fractures in Elderly Patients. *J. Bone Jt. Surg. Am.* **2013**, *95*, 2050–2055. [CrossRef]
8. Fraser, A.N.; Bjørdal, J.; Wagle, T.M.; Karlberg, A.C.; Lien, O.A.; Eilertsen, L.; Mader, K.; Apold, H.; Larsen, L.B.; Madsen, J.E.; et al. Reverse Shoulder Arthroplasty Is Superior to Plate Fixation at 2 Years for Displaced Proximal Humeral Fractures in the Elderly: A Multicenter Randomized Controlled Trial. *J. Bone Jt. Surg. Am.* **2020**, *102*, 477–485. [CrossRef]
9. Dillon, M.T.; Prentice, H.A.; Burfeind, W.E.; Chan, P.H.; Navarro, R.A. The Increasing Role of Reverse Total Shoulder Arthroplasty in the Treatment of Proximal Humerus Fractures. *Injury* **2019**, *50*, 676–680. [CrossRef]

10. Zyto, K. Non-Operative Treatment of Comminuted Fractures of the Proximal Humerus in Elderly Patients. *Injury* **1998**, *29*, 349–352. [CrossRef]
11. Clement, N.D.; Aitken, S.A.; Duckworth, A.D.; McQueen, M.M.; Court-Brown, C.M. The Outcome of Fractures in Very Elderly Patients. *J. Bone Jt. Surg. Br. Vol.* **2011**, *93-B*, 806–810. [CrossRef]
12. Moher, D.; Liberati, A.; Tetzlaff, J.; Altman, D.G. Preferred Reporting Items for Systematic Reviews and Meta-Analyses: The Prisma Statement. *PLoS Med.* **2009**, *6*, e1000097. [CrossRef] [PubMed]
13. Stroup, D.F.; Berlin, J.A.; Morton, S.C.; Olkin, I.; Williamson, G.D.; Rennie, D.; Moher, D.; Becker, B.J.; Sipe, T.A.; Thacker, S.B.; et al. Meta-Analysis of Observational Studies in Epidemiologya Proposal for Reporting. *JAMA* **2000**, *283*, 2008–2012. [CrossRef] [PubMed]
14. Lopiz, Y.; Alcobía-Díaz, B.; Galán-Olleros, M.; García-Fernández, C.; Picado, A.L.; Marco, F. Reverse Shoulder Arthroplasty Versus Nonoperative Treatment for 3- or 4-Part Proximal Humeral Fractures in Elderly Patients: A Prospective Randomized Controlled Trial. *J. Shoulder Elb. Surg.* **2019**, *28*, 2259–2271. [CrossRef] [PubMed]
15. Chivot, M.; Lami, D.; Bizzozero, P.; Galland, A.; Argenson, J.-N. Three- and Four-Part Displaced Proximal Humeral Fractures in Patients Older Than 70 Years: Reverse Shoulder Arthroplasty or Nonsurgical Treatment? *J. Shoulder Elb. Surg.* **2019**, *28*, 252–259. [CrossRef]
16. Roberson, T.A.; Granade, C.M.; Hunt, Q.; Griscom, J.T.; Adams, K.J.; Momaya, A.M.; Kwapisz, A.; Kissenberth, M.J.; Tolan, S.J.; Hawkins, R.J.; et al. Nonoperative Management Versus Reverse Shoulder Arthroplasty for Treatment of 3- and 4-Part Proximal Humeral Fractures in Older Adults. *J. Shoulder Elb. Surg.* **2017**, *26*, 1017–1022. [CrossRef]
17. Grassi, F.A.; Zorzolo, I. Reverse Shoulder Arthroplasty without Subscapularis Repair for the Treatment of Proximal Humeral Fractures in the Elderly. *Musculoskelet. Surg.* **2014**, *98* (Suppl. 1), 5–13. [CrossRef]
18. Grubhofer, F.; Wieser, K.; Meyer, D.C.; Catanzaro, S.; Beeler, S.; Riede, U.; Gerber, C. Reverse Total Shoulder Arthroplasty for Acute Head-Splitting, 3- and 4-Part Fractures of the Proximal Humerus in the Elderly. *J. Shoulder Elb. Surg.* **2016**, *25*, 1690–1698. [CrossRef] [PubMed]
19. Klein, M.; Juschka, M.; Hinkenjann, B.; Scherger, B.; Ostermann, P.A. Treatment of Comminuted Fractures of the Proximal Humerus in Elderly Patients with the Delta Iii Reverse Shoulder Prosthesis. *J. Orthop. Trauma* **2008**, *22*, 698–704. [CrossRef]
20. Klug, A.; Harth, J.; Hoffmann, R.; Gramlich, Y. Surgical Treatment of Complex Proximal Humeral Fractures in Elderly Patients: A Matched-Pair Analysis of Angular-Stable Plating Vs. Reverse Shoulder Arthroplasty. *J. Shoulder Elb. Surg.* **2020**, *29*, 1796–1803. [CrossRef]
21. Lenarz, C.; Shishani, Y.; McCrum, C.; Nowinski, R.J.; Edwards, T.B.; Gobezie, R. Is Reverse Shoulder Arthroplasty Appropriate for the Treatment of Fractures in the Older Patient? Early Observations. *Clin. Orthop. Relat. Res.* **2011**, *469*, 3324–3331. [CrossRef]
22. Lopiz, Y.; García-Coiradas, J.; Serrano-Mateo, L.; García-Fernández, C.; Marco, F. Reverse Shoulder Arthroplasty for Acute Proximal Humeral Fractures in the Geriatric Patient: Results, Health-Related Quality of Life and Complication Rates. *Int. Orthop.* **2016**, *40*, 771–781. [CrossRef]
23. Luciani, P.; Farinelli, L.; Procaccini, R.; Verducci, C.; Gigante, A. Primary Reverse Shoulder Arthroplasty for Acute Proximal Humerus Fractures: A 5-Year Long Term Retrospective Study of Elderly Patients. *Injury* **2019**, *50*, 1974–1977. [CrossRef]
24. Ohl, X.; Bonnevialle, N.; Gallinet, D.; Ramdane, N.; Valenti, P.; Decroocq, L.; Boileau, P. How the Greater Tuberosity Affects Clinical Outcomes after Reverse Shoulder Arthroplasty for Proximal Humeral Fractures. *J. Shoulder Elb. Surg.* **2018**, *27*, 2139–2144. [CrossRef] [PubMed]
25. Repetto, I.; Alessio-Mazzola, M.; Cerruti, P.; Sanguineti, F.; Formica, M.; Felli, L. Surgical Management of Complex Proximal Humeral Fractures: Pinning, Locked Plate and Arthroplasty: Clinical Results and Functional Outcome on Retrospective Series of Patients. *Musculoskelet. Surg.* **2017**, *101*, 153–158. [CrossRef] [PubMed]
26. Schmalzl, J.; Jessen, M.; Holschen, M.; Cohen, B.C.; Steinbeck, J.; Lehmann, L.-J.; Denard, P.J. Tuberosity Healing Improves Functional Outcome Following Primary Reverse Shoulder Arthroplasty for Proximal Humeral Fractures with a 135° Prosthesis. *Eur. J. Orthop. Surg. Traumatol.* **2020**, *30*, 909–916. [CrossRef]
27. Baudi, P.; Campochiaro, G.; Serafini, F.; Gazzotti, G.; Matino, G.; Rovesta, C.; Catani, F. Hemiarthroplasty Versus Reverse Shoulder Arthroplasty: Comparative Study of Functional and Radiological Outcomes in the Treatment of Acute Proximal Humerus Fracture. *Musculoskelet. Surg.* **2014**, *98* (Suppl. 1), 19–25. [CrossRef] [PubMed]
28. Sebastiá-Forcada, E.; Cebrián-Gómez, R.; Lizaur-Utrilla, A.; Gil-Guillén, V. Reverse Shoulder Arthroplasty Versus Hemiarthroplasty for Acute Proximal Humeral Fractures. A Blinded, Randomized, Controlled, Prospective Study. *J. Shoulder Elb. Surg.* **2014**, *23*, 1419–1426. [CrossRef]
29. Simovitch, R.W.; Roche, C.P.; Jones, R.B.; Routman, H.D.; Marczuk, Y.; Wright, T.W.; Zuckerman, J.D. Effect of Tuberosity Healing on Clinical Outcomes in Elderly Patients Treated with a Reverse Shoulder Arthroplasty for 3- and 4-Part Proximal Humerus Fractures. *J. Orthop. Trauma* **2019**, *33*, e39–e45. [CrossRef]
30. Solomon, J.A.; Joseph, S.M.; Shishani, Y.; Victoroff, B.N.; Wilber, J.H.; Gobezie, R.; Gillespie, R.J. Cost Analysis of Hemiarthroplasty Versus Reverse Shoulder Arthroplasty for Fractures. *Orthopedics* **2016**, *39*, 230–234. [CrossRef]
31. Torrens, C.; Alentorn-Geli, E.; Mingo, F.; Gamba, C.; Santana, F. Reverse Shoulder Arthroplasty for the Treatment of Acute Complex Proximal Humeral Fractures: Influence of Greater Tuberosity Healing on the Functional Outcomes. *J. Orthop. Surg.* **2018**, *26*, 2309499018760132. [CrossRef] [PubMed]

32. Valenti, P.; Katz, D.; Kilinc, A.; Elkholti, K.; Gasiunas, V. Mid-Term Outcome of Reverse Shoulder Prostheses in Complex Proximal Humeral Fractures. *Acta Orthop. Belg.* **2012**, *78*, 442–449.
33. van der Merwe, M.; Boyle, M.J.; Frampton, C.M.A.; Ball, C.M. Reverse Shoulder Arthroplasty Compared with Hemiarthroplasty in the Treatment of Acute Proximal Humeral Fractures. *J. Shoulder Elb. Surg.* **2017**, *26*, 1539–1545. [CrossRef] [PubMed]
34. Wolfensperger, F.; Grüninger, P.; Dietrich, M.; Völlink, M.; Benninger, E.; Schläppi, M.; Meier, C. Reverse Shoulder Arthroplasty for Complex Fractures of the Proximal Humerus in Elderly Patients: Impact on the Level of Independency, Early Function, and Pain Medication. *J. Shoulder Elb. Surg.* **2017**, *26*, 1462–1468. [CrossRef] [PubMed]
35. Wright, J.O.; Ho, A.; Kalma, J.; Koueiter, D.; Esterle, J.; Marcantonio, D.; Wiater, J.M.; Wiater, B. Uncemented Reverse Total Shoulder Arthroplasty as Initial Treatment for Comminuted Proximal Humerus Fractures. *J. Orthop. Trauma* **2019**, *33*, e263–e269. [CrossRef] [PubMed]
36. Young, S.W.; Segal, B.S.; Turner, P.C.; Poon, P.C. Comparison of Functional Outcomes of Reverse Shoulder Arthroplasty Versus Hemiarthroplasty in the Primary Treatment of Acute Proximal Humerus Fracture. *ANZ J. Surg.* **2010**, *80*, 789–793. [CrossRef] [PubMed]
37. Bogner, R.; Resch, H.; Moroder, P. Functional and Quality-of-Life Results of Displaced and Nondisplaced Proximal Humeral Fractures Treated Conservatively. *J. Orthop. Trauma* **2014**, *28*, e178. [CrossRef] [PubMed]
38. Bonnevialle, N.; Tournier, C.; Clavert, P.; Ohl, X.; Sirveaux, F.; Saragaglia, D. Hemiarthroplasty Versus Reverse Shoulder Arthroplasty in 4-Part Displaced Fractures of the Proximal Humerus: Multicenter Retrospective Study. *Orthop. Traumatol. Surg. Res.* **2016**, *102*, 569–573. [CrossRef]
39. Boyle, M.J.; Youn, S.-M.; Frampton, C.M.A.; Ball, C.M. Functional Outcomes of Reverse Shoulder Arthroplasty Compared with Hemiarthroplasty for Acute Proximal Humeral Fractures. *J. Shoulder Elb. Surg.* **2013**, *22*, 32–37. [CrossRef]
40. Cazeneuve, J.F.; Cristofari, D.J. The Reverse Shoulder Prosthesis in the Treatment of Fractures of the Proximal Humerus in the Elderly. *J. Bone Jt. Surg. Br.* **2010**, *92*, 535–539. [CrossRef]
41. Gallinet, D.; Cazeneuve, J.F.; Boyer, E.; Menu, G.; Obert, L.; Ohl, X.; Bonnevialle, N.; Valenti, P.; Boileau, P. Reverse Shoulder Arthroplasty for Recent Proximal Humerus Fractures: Outcomes in 422 Cases. *Orthop. Traumatol. Surg. Res.* **2019**, *105*, 805–811. [CrossRef] [PubMed]
42. Garrigues, G.E.; Johnston, P.S.; Pepe, M.D.; Tucker, B.S.; Ramsey, M.L.; Austin, L.S. Hemiarthroplasty Versus Reverse Total Shoulder Arthroplasty for Acute Proximal Humerus Fractures in Elderly Patients. *Orthopedics* **2012**, *35*, e703–e708. [CrossRef] [PubMed]
43. Barbosa, L.; Pires, L.; Rego, P.; Alonso, R. Reverse Total Shoulder Arthroplasty for Treatment of 3- and 4-Part Proximal Humeral Fractures: Clinical and Radiological Analysis with Minimum Follow-up of 2 Years. *Geriatr. Orthop. Surg. Rehabil.* **2020**, *11*, 2151459320915321. [CrossRef] [PubMed]
44. Boons, H.W.; Goosen, J.H.; van Grinsven, S.; van Susante, J.L.; van Loon, C.J. Hemiarthroplasty for Humeral Four-Part Fractures for Patients 65 Years and Older: A Randomized Controlled Trial. *Clin. Orthop. Relat. Res.* **2012**, *470*, 3483–3491. [CrossRef] [PubMed]
45. Brouwer, M.E.; Reininga, I.H.F.; El Moumni, M.; Wendt, K.W. Outcomes of Operative and Nonoperative Treatment of 3- and 4-Part Proximal Humeral Fractures in Elderly: A 10-Year Retrospective Cohort Study. *Eur. J. Trauma. Emerg. Surg.* **2019**, *45*, 131–138. [CrossRef] [PubMed]
46. Clement, N.D.; Duckworth, A.D.; McQueen, M.M.; Court-Brown, C.M. The Outcome of Proximal Humeral Fractures in the Elderly: Predictors of Mortality and Function. *Bone Jt. J.* **2014**, *96-B*, 970–977. [CrossRef] [PubMed]
47. Rangan, A.; Handoll, H.; Brealey, S.; Jefferson, L.; Keding, A.; Martin, B.C.; Goodchild, L.; Chuang, L.H.; Hewitt, C.; Torgerson, D. Surgical vs. Nonsurgical Treatment of Adults with Displaced Fractures of the Proximal Humerus: The Profher Randomized Clinical Trial. *JAMA* **2015**, *313*, 1037–1047. [CrossRef] [PubMed]
48. Dezfuli, B.; King, J.J.; Farmer, K.W.; Struk, A.M.; Wright, T.W. Outcomes of Reverse Total Shoulder Arthroplasty as Primary Versus Revision Procedure for Proximal Humerus Fractures. *J. Shoulder Elb. Surg.* **2016**, *25*, 1133–1137. [CrossRef] [PubMed]
49. Panagopoulos, G.N.; Pugliese, M.; Leonidou, A.; Butt, F.; Jaibaji, M.; Megaloikonomos, P.D.; Consigliere, P.; Sforza, G.; Atoun, E.; Levy, O. Acute Versus Delayed Reverse Total Shoulder Arthroplasty for Proximal Humeral Fractures: A Consecutive Cohort Study. *J. Shoulder Elb. Surg.* **2022**, *31*, 276–285. [CrossRef]
50. Kang, J.R.; Dubiel, M.J.; Cofield, R.H.; Steinmann, S.P.; Elhassan, B.T.; Morrey, M.E.; Sperling, J.W.; Sanchez-Sotelo, J. Primary Reverse Shoulder Arthroplasty Using Contemporary Implants Is Associated with Very Low Reoperation Rates. *J. Shoulder Elb. Surg.* **2019**, *28*, S175–S180. [CrossRef]
51. Simovitch, R.; Flurin, P.-H.; Wright, T.; Zuckerman, J.D.; Roche, C.P. Quantifying Success after Total Shoulder Arthroplasty: The Minimal Clinically Important Difference. *J. Shoulder Elb. Surg.* **2018**, *27*, 298–305. [CrossRef]
52. Wijgman, A.J.; Roolker, W.; Patt, T.W.; Raaymakers, E.L.F.B.; Marti, R.K. Open Reduction and Internal Fixation of Three and Four-Part Fractures of the Proximal Part of the Humerus. *JBJS* **2002**, *84*, 1919–1925. [CrossRef]
53. Bacle, G.; Nové-Josserand, L.; Garaud, P.; Walch, G. Long-Term Outcomes of Reverse Total Shoulder Arthroplasty: A Follow-up of a Previous Study. *J. Bone Jt. Surg. Am.* **2017**, *99*, 454–461. [CrossRef] [PubMed]
54. Ascione, F.; Domos, P.; Guarrella, V.; Chelli, M.; Boileau, P.; Walch, G. Long-Term Humeral Complications after Grammont-Style Reverse Shoulder Arthroplasty. *J. Shoulder Elb. Surg.* **2018**, *27*, 1065–1071. [CrossRef]

55. United Nations. *World Population Prospects 2019: Highlights*; United Nations, Department of Economic and Social Affairs Population Division: New York, NY, USA, 2019.
56. Polinder, S.; Haagsma, J.; Panneman, M.; Scholten, A.; Brugmans, M.; Van Beeck, E. The Economic Burden of Injury: Health Care and Productivity Costs of Injuries in the Netherlands. *Accid. Anal. Prev.* **2016**, *93*, 92–100. [CrossRef] [PubMed]
57. Erixon, F.; van der Marel, E. *What Is Driving the Rise in Health Care Expenditures? An Inquiry into the Nature and Causes of the Cost Disease*; European Centre for International Political Economy: Brussels, Belgium, 2011.
58. Abdel Khalik, H.; Humphries, B.; Zoratti, M.; Axelrod, D.; Kruse, C.; Ristevski, B.; Rajaratnam, K.; Gardner, M.; Tarride, J.-E. Johal, H. Reverse Total Shoulder Arthroplasty Is the Most Cost-Effective Treatment Strategy for Proximal Humerus Fractures in Older Adults: A Cost-Utility Analysis. *Clin. Orthop. Relat. Res.* **2022**, *480*, 2013–2026. [CrossRef]

Journal of
Clinical Medicine

MDPI

Article

Palliative Non-Operative Management in Geriatric Hip Fracture Patients: When Would Surgeons Abstain from Surgery?

Michael Bui [1,*], Catharina G. M. Groothuis-Oudshoorn [1], Annemieke Witteveen [2] and Johannes H. Hegeman [2,3,*]

[1] Department of Health Technology and Services Research, Technical Medical Centre, University of Twente, 7500 AE Enschede, The Netherlands; c.g.m.oudshoorn@utwente.nl

[2] Department of Biomedical Signals and Systems, Technical Medical Centre, University of Twente, 7500 AE Enschede, The Netherlands; a.witteveen@utwente.nl

[3] Department of Surgery, Ziekenhuisgroep Twente, 7609 PP Almelo, The Netherlands

* Correspondence: m.bui@utwente.nl (M.B.); h.hegeman@zgt.nl (J.H.H.); Tel.: +31-088-708-5233 (J.H.H.)

Abstract: Background: For hip fracture patients with a limited life expectancy, operative and palliative non-operative management (P-NOM) can yield similar quality of life outcomes. However, evidence on when to abstain from surgery is lacking. The aim of this study was to quantify the influence of patient characteristics on surgeons' decisions to recommend P-NOM. **Methods:** Dutch surgical residents and orthopaedic trauma surgeons were enrolled in a conjoint analysis and structured expert judgement (SEJ). The participants assessed 16 patient cases comprising 10 clinically relevant characteristics. For each case, they recommended either surgery or P-NOM and estimated the 30-day postoperative mortality risk. Treatment recommendations were analysed using Bayesian logistic regression, and perceived risks were pooled with equal and performance-based weights using Cooke's Classical Model. **Results:** The conjoint analysis and SEJ were completed by 14 and 9 participants, respectively. Participants were more likely to recommend P-NOM to patients with metastatic carcinomas (OR: 4.42, CrI: 2.14–8.95), severe heart failure (OR: 4.05, CrI: 1.89–8.29), end-stage renal failure (OR: 3.54, CrI: 1.76–7.35) and dementia (OR: 3.35, CrI: 1.70–7.06). The patient receiving the most P-NOM recommendations (12/14) had a pooled perceived risk of 30-day mortality between 50.8 and 62.7%. **Conclusions:** Overall, comorbidities had the strongest influence on participants' decisions to recommend P-NOM. Nevertheless, practice variation and heterogeneity in risk perceptions were substantial. Hence, more decision support for considering P-NOM is needed.

Keywords: hip fractures; geriatrics; frailty; palliative non-operative management; decision-making; conjoint analysis; structured expert judgement

1. Introduction

In worldwide practice, operative treatment is considered to be superior over non-operative management in terms of clinical outcomes for the majority of hip fracture patients [1,2]. It is well established that the mortality rate is significantly higher in non-operatively treated patients than in operatively treated patients [3–5]. However, in the case of frail older adults with a limited life expectancy, surgeons have started to question the superiority of surgery [6,7]. Clinical guidelines often focus on functional recovery to pre-fracture levels [8], while patients with a limited life expectancy might prioritise their quality of life (QoL) instead [9]. In these cases, surgical overtreatment should be avoided due to its negative repercussions on patients and families, which include iatrogenesis and anxiety [10,11]. Hence, there is increasing awareness that palliative non-operative management (P-NOM) should be considered as a valid care option amongst frail older adults [7,9,12–15].

Particularly amongst patients of advanced age with multiple physical and cognitive comorbidities, there is a pressing need for counselling regarding survival prognoses and advance care planning [16]. By properly informing frail patients on the available treatment options and examining how these align with their goals of care through shared decision-making (SDM) [17], patients and clinicians might come to the conclusion that P-NOM is preferred. Affirmatively, a single-centre retrospective cohort study found that the percentage of patients electing P-NOM increased significantly over the years (2.7% vs. 9.1%) after implementing comprehensive geriatric assessments with SDM [18]. Still, uncertainties regarding the optimal treatment choice might persist during SDM in complex patient cases [7]. A paucity of decision support for P-NOM in current clinical guidelines poses challenges for the preoperative decision-making process. Therefore, more evidence regarding the choice between surgery and P-NOM is required to optimise treatment plans for frail older adults.

Only a few studies have thus far investigated the motives behind electing P-NOM. In most cases, P-NOM was preferred when early mortality or other poor prognoses were anticipated for operative treatment due to frailty, for example, caused by comorbidities, poor functional status and declining cognitive functioning [18,19]. While these attributes could be used to identify patients who would not benefit from operative treatment, it remains a challenging task. Various prediction models for 30-day mortality following hip fracture surgery have been developed to identify patients who are unfit for operative treatment [20–24]. However, these models showcased moderate discriminative ability, making them premature for clinical practice. When data-driven approaches are not sufficiently reliable, domain experts should be consulted [25,26]. The synthesis of clinicians' treatment preferences for various patient cases aids in understanding which specific patients would benefit from which treatments [27].

The current study proposes a clinical vignette methodology to elicit and analyse surgical residents' and orthopaedic trauma surgeons' treatment preferences for frail older hip fracture patients with limited life expectancy. This is a type of conjoint analysis (CA) [28,29], in which the decision-making behaviours of medical experts are studied in various scenarios known as vignettes [30]. A vignette is defined as "a short, carefully constructed description of a person, object, or situation, representing a systematic combination of characteristics" [31] (p. 128). Given that clinicians' judgements of vignettes and their responses to real-life cases are sufficiently congruent [32], clinical vignette studies provide a means to reliably simulate and analyse complex decision-making processes in healthcare. The insights gained facilitate the understanding of which factors are influential in decision-making for surgeons and help inform clinical practices and policy development to support decision-making [33].

While individual patient attributes may influence physicians' treatment preferences, they may also shape their overall perception of patients' early mortality risks. Capturing early mortality risk assessments is pertinent since they could influence the likelihood of considering P-NOM [6–8]. Therefore, the current study proposes to additionally elicit the perceived risks of 30-day postoperative death for each vignette through a structured expert judgement (SEJ) [34].

To support preoperative decision-making for frail hip fracture patients with a limited life expectancy, it is imperative to understand how patient characteristics and mortality risk perceptions affect treatment decisions. Hence, the aim of this exploratory study is to conduct a clinical vignette study and SEJ to systematically capture the expertise of surgical residents and orthopaedic trauma surgeons to synthesise recommendations for clinical guidelines. To the best of our knowledge, we are the first to conduct a clinical vignette study and SEJ to examine preoperative decision-making for frail hip fracture patients.

2. Materials and Methods

2.1. Data Collection

The clinical vignette study and SEJ were distributed to surgical residents and orthopaedic trauma surgeons from three Dutch hospitals through an online survey between June and August 2022. Participants were approached through an e-mail explaining the purpose of the study along with a link to the survey.

2.2. Selection of Patient Attributes and Levels for the Vignettes

Predictors for early mortality were chosen as primary attributes for the design of the vignettes, since P-NOM was mostly reserved for patients with a limited life expectancy [8,9]. In our previous work [35], we conducted a systematic review and meta-analysis to identify these predictors. To analyse participants' decision-making behaviours as comprehensively as possible, the vignettes were designed using the maximum number of attributes recommended in practice, that is, 10 attributes [33].

All high-quality evidence predictors for 30-day mortality identified in our meta-analysis were selected as attributes for the vignettes (age, gender, ASA classification [36], institutional residence and metastatic cancer). Amongst the moderate-quality evidence predictors, only those for which confidence in the existence of a true significant association with mortality was expressed were selected (dementia, renal failure and heart failure). To increase ecological validity, functional status was included, as guidelines for preoperative decision-making are centred around functional recovery [9]. Finally, to enforce applicability to the study population of interest, fracture type was selected as an attribute.

When constructing vignettes, implausible combinations of attribute levels should be avoided. Amongst the chosen attributes, implausibility concerns were raised for the ASA score. Since ASA scores increase with the severity of diseases, not all pairs of comorbidities and ASA scores would be logical to present simultaneously in the vignettes. Hence, attribute levels of comorbidities were defined such that they were maximally compatible with all ASA attribute levels chosen in this study. To keep the total number of vignettes low, the number of attribute levels was mostly restricted to two. Since a dichotomy of health conditions and functional statuses could potentially be too coarse to inform decision-making, the vignettes were pilot tested with a surgical resident and orthopaedic trauma surgeon. Both physicians agreed that it was not necessary to introduce additional attribute levels. An overview of the attribute levels along with the rationale behind the chosen definitions is depicted in Table 1.

Table 1. Overview of attributes and their levels as presented to the participants in the vignettes. For each attribute level, the rationale behind the chosen definition is provided.

Attribute	Levels	Rationale
Age	The patient is in the age group 80–89 years The patient is 90 years or older	80 years was chosen as a lower bound, based on the average age of hip fracture patients. The cut-off between the two levels was based on the observation that complication risks and mortality rates differed significantly between octogenarians and nonagenarians [37].
Gender	The patient is female The patient is male	-
Fracture type	The patient has an undisplaced femoral neck fracture The patient has a displaced femoral neck fracture The patient has an extracapsular fracture	The invasiveness of the required surgical intervention differs between displaced and undisplaced femoral neck fractures. Most extracapsular fractures are treated with intramedullary nails in The Netherlands. Hence, extracapsular fractures were not further distinguished.
Physical status	The patient has severe systemic diseases without a constant threat to life (ASA III) The patient has severe systemic diseases with a constant threat to life (ASA IV)	It was anticipated that ASA I, II and V would not require decision support: all ASA I and II patients would be treated operatively [8], and all ASA V patients would be treated non-operatively.
Severe heart failure	The patient has no severe heart failure (LVEF $\geq$ 30%) The patient has severe heart failure (LVEF < 30%)	A moderate-to-severe reduction in left ventricular ejection fraction (LVEF) is congruent with both ASA III and IV [38,39]. The corresponding cut-off of <30% was based on [40].
Metastatic carcinoma	The patient has no metastatic carcinomas The patient has metastatic carcinomas	The presence of non-metastatic cancer only increases the 30-day mortality risk weakly [35]. Hence, patients without metastases were not further distinguished into cancer-free and non-metastatic cancer patients.

Table 1. *Cont.*

Attribute	Levels	Rationale
End-stage renal failure	The patient has no end-stage renal failure requiring dialysis The patient has end-stage renal failure requiring dialysis	The dialysis requirement complies with both the ASA III and ASA IV classifications [38,39]. Due to the high prevalence of renal failure amongst adults aged ≥80 years [41], no distinction was made between mild renal failure and the absence of renal failure.
Preoperative residence	The patient lived at home prior to admission The patient lived in a care institution prior to admission	-
Functional status *	The patient has no severe functional handicaps (Katz 3–6) The patient has severe functional handicaps (Katz 0–2)	Low pre-fracture functioning was a common reason for choosing non-operative treatment [9,18]. Hence, the extreme end of the Katz scale was chosen.
Dementia	The patient has no dementia The patient has dementia	Dementia is a well-known predictor of postoperative delirium [42–44]. A single level for dementia was thus thought to be sufficient to influence clinicians' decisions.

* Participants were provided with a link to a document where the Katz scores were explained in more detail, where 0 was defined as completely dependent and 6 as functionally independent.

2.3. Experimental Design of Patient Vignettes

The 10 attributes yielded a full factorial design comprising $2^9 \times 3 = 1536$ vignettes. However, one attribute level combination was deemed implausible: ASA III paired with metastatic cancer [45]. Hence, all vignettes containing this combination were removed from the full factorial design to reduce measurement errors [46], leaving a total of 1152 vignettes. As it was not feasible to present all 1152 vignettes to each participant, a D-optimal main effects design [47] was generated from this subset with R version 4.0.2 using the skpr package [48]. Through experimental designs, smaller subsets of vignettes can be selected while safeguarding the precision and unbiasedness of the statistical analysis [49]. The number of vignettes was minimised by inspecting the relative gain in D-efficiency upon increasing the number of vignettes over a range of 12 to 24. Based on these trials, a design comprising 16 vignettes with a D-efficiency of 94.4% was chosen. The full experimental design can be found in Table A1 of Appendix A.

2.4. Survey Design

The survey consisted of four sections. The first section covered background questions about participants' medical professional status and years of working experience. In the second section, they were presented with the vignettes. For each vignette, they were asked to (1) recommend either surgery or P-NOM, (2) rate how certain they were about the optimality of their recommendation on a 5-point Likert scale and (3) estimate the probability of 30-day postoperative mortality. Whenever they elected operative treatment, they were asked whether the treatment intentions were palliative or curative. In the third section, participants answered 14 SEJ questions to assess their expertise in mortality prediction. Finally, participants gave feedback on information they missed in the vignettes.

2.5. Elicitation and Analysis of Treatment Preferences

The aim of the vignette study was to quantify the average impact of patient attributes on participants' treatment preferences in terms of odds ratios (ORs). ORs were estimated using a hierarchical Bayesian logit with random intercepts, in which treatment choices were regressed against the attributes in the vignettes. To examine the degree to which treatment recommendations could be explained by participants' personal preferences rather than changes in attribute levels, the intraclass correlation coefficient (ICC) was computed.

A Bayesian estimation framework was chosen for the main analysis since a low response rate to the survey was anticipated. When prior knowledge about the effect sizes of the individual attributes is available, Bayesian models can still provide valid regression outcomes despite small sample sizes [50–54]. Since early mortality risk is the primary reason for electing P-NOM [8], we assumed that the attributes' prognostic values for death could be seen as proxies for participants' inclinations to choose P-NOM. Therefore, we primarily used our systematic review and meta-analysis for predictors of early mortality to derive prior knowledge on the effect sizes and uncertainties around the beta coefficients of the Bayesian model (see Table 2). We followed the When-to-Worry-and-How-to-Avoid-the-Misuse-of-Bayesian-Statistics checklist to ensure methodological rigour [55].

Table 2. Overview of prior specifications expressed on a logarithmic scale. All betas denote log odds ratios (ORs).

Parameter	Distribution	Specification	Prior Type	Background Knowledge
β_0	Normal	N(−2.75, 1)	Weakly informative	Here, 3% of the Dutch patients are treated non-operatively [56]. As the vignettes exclude ASA I-II, β_0 was expected to be slightly higher. The prior yields a mean probability of 6.0% (95% CrI: 0.9–31.2%) in favour of P-NOM for the null model.
β_{gender}	Normal	N(0.09, 1)	Weakly informative	Male gender is a high-quality evidence predictor for 30-day mortality [35]. However, it was deemed unlikely that this would be reflected in participants' treatment preferences. Hence, the informativeness of the prior was decreased, yielding a mean OR of 1.1 (95% CrI: 0.15–7.80) in favour of P-NOM.
$\beta_{extracapsular}$	Normal	N(0.09, 1)	Weakly informative	Compared to undisplaced femoral neck fractures, extracapsular fractures have a higher postoperative anaemia incidence [57]. Due to the lack of strong evidence for increased mortality risk [58], a small mean OR of 1.1 (95% CrI: 0.15–7.80) in favour of P-NOM was assumed.
β_{DFN}	Normal	N(0.18, 1)	Weakly informative	Displaced femoral neck fractures require more invasive surgical intervention than their undisplaced counterparts. As quantitative evidence was lacking, a small mean OR of 1.2 (95% CrI: 0.17–8.51) in favour of P-NOM was assumed.
β_{ASA}	Normal	N(0.69, 1)	Informative	ASA scores increase 30-day mortality risk with an OR of 2.62 (95% CI: 2.21–3.12) per point increase [35]. During the vignette study pilot test, a surgical resident expressed indifference towards ASA scores due to the subjectivity of the scoring system. A relatively wide prior was chosen to reflect uncertainty in the influence of ASA scores, with a mean OR of 2.0 (95% CrI: 0.5–7.99) in favour of P-NOM.
β_{heart}	Normal	N(0.69, 0.5)	Informative	Heart failure increases the risk of 30-day mortality with an OR of 2.18 (95% CI: 1.25–3.82) [35]. The prior yields a mean OR of 2.0 (95% CrI: 0.50–7.98) in favour of P-NOM.
$\beta_{metastasis}$	Normal	N(0.92, 0.3)	Informative	Metastasis increases the 30-day mortality risk with an OR of 2.83 (95% CI: 2.58–3.10) [35]. The informativeness of the prior was increased due to the high quality of the evidence and the narrow CI width. The prior yields a mean OR of 2.5 (95% CrI: 0.85–7.32) in favour of P-NOM.
β_{ESRF}	Normal	N(0.79, 0.5)	Informative	Chronic renal failure increases the risk of 30-day mortality with an OR of 1.61 (95% CI: 1.11–2.34) [35]. The risk is even higher for ESRF (95% CI: 3.57–12.58) [59]. The prior yields a mean OR of 2.2 (95% CrI: 0.55–8.81) in favour of P-NOM.
$\beta_{institution}$	Normal	N(0.47, 0.5)	Informative	Institutional residence increases the risk of 30-day mortality with an OR of 1.81 (95% CI: 1.31–2.49) [35]. The prior yields a mean OR of 1.6 (95% CrI: 0.40–6.42) in favour of P-NOM.
$\beta_{functional}$	Normal	N(0.47, 0.7)	Informative	The effect size of severe functional handicaps was assumed to be similar to that of institutional residence. However, due to the lack of quantitative evidence, a slightly wider prior was specified with a mean OR of 1.6 (95% CrI: 0.31–8.26).
$\beta_{dementia}$	Normal	N(0.34, 0.5)	Informative	Dementia increases the risk of 30-day mortality with an OR of 1.57 (95% CI: 1.30–1.90) [35]. The prior yields a mean OR of 1.4 (95% CrI: 0.35–5.60) in favour of P-NOM.
u_i	Normal	$N(0, \sigma^2_u)$	Uninformative	N/A
σ^2_u	Inverse Wishart	IW(1, 1)	Uninformative	N/A
$\varepsilon_{i,j}$	Multivariate normal	MVN(0, I) [1]	Uninformative	N/A

DFN displaced femoral neck fracture, ASA American Society of Anesthesiologists physical status classification, ESRF end-stage renal failure, u_i random intercept term for a single participant, σ^2_u variance of u_i, $\varepsilon_{i,j}$ random error term for a single participant and vignette, CrI credible interval. [1] Multivariate normal distribution with the mean vector equal to the zero vector and the covariance matrix equal to the identity matrix.

The posterior distributions for each regression coefficient were estimated via Markov Chain Monte Carlo (MCMC) sampling [60]. For this, 15,000 posterior samples were drawn after a burn-in phase of 1000 samples. Point estimates were obtained by computing the posterior means. The model was implemented in R version 4.0.2, using the MCMCpack package [61].

2.6. Bayesian Convergence Diagnostics and Sensitivity Analysis

To ensure that the regression coefficients had converged to stable estimates, several diagnostic tests were conducted. First, trace and autocorrelation plots were inspected for MCMC convergence. The stationarity of the Markov chains was assessed with Geweke's convergence test [62]. Second, to determine whether the resulting posteriors were sufficiently smooth, histograms of the posterior draws were inspected.

Finally, to assess the extent to which our prior beliefs affected the ORs, the regression analysis was re-evaluated with noninformative priors, that is, N(0, 2), which neither favoured P-NOM nor surgery. The influence of priors was considered (1) small if the relative deviation (RD) was at most 10% and the substantive results remained the same, (2) moderate if 10% < RD $\leq$ 20% and the substantive results remained the same and (3) large otherwise.

$$RD = 100\% \times |OR_{informative} - OR_{uninformative}| / OR_{informative} \quad (1)$$

2.7. A Priori Power Analysis and Sample Size Calculations

Health policy recommendations based on non-significant outcomes should not be made without considering whether the study had sufficient power to detect small yet meaningful effects [63]. Therefore, an a priori power analysis was conducted using 10,000 Monte Carlo simulations [64]. For simplicity, a logit model was used as an analytical outcome model in the simulations to obtain a rough estimate for the required sample size. The resulting power curves shown in Figure 1 indicated that approximately 55 participants were required to attain a power above 60% for 8/11 attribute levels.

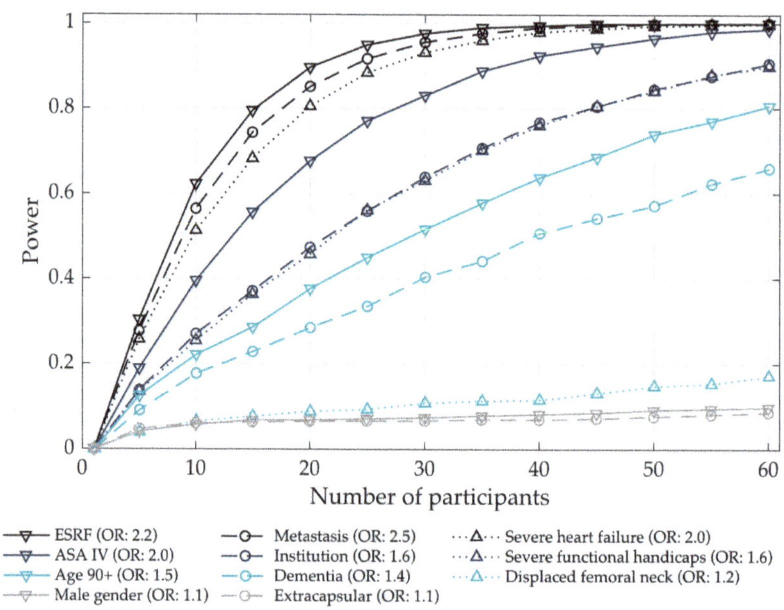

Figure 1. Power curves for the attribute levels used in the vignettes. The respective odds ratios (ORs), which were assumed during the power calculations, are listed behind each attribute level.

2.8. Elicitation and Analysis of Risk Perceptions

The goal of the SEJ was to elicit and aggregate participants' 30-day mortality risk perceptions of frail geriatric patients undergoing hip fracture surgery. Expert elicitation was performed using Cooke's Classical Model for SEJs [34]. The Classical Model enforces empirical control by first scoring how statistically accurate and informative participants are in the estimation of verifiable variables, prior to aggregating their judgements on unknown variables. Participants with higher scores are assigned higher performance-based weights in the aggregation to obtain the best estimate of the unknown target variable.

Calibration questions were used to measure participants' performances. In this case, calibration questions referred to verifiable questions about 30-day mortality prevalence percentages amongst subpopulations of hip fracture patients. Participants are not expected to know the exact percentages but should be able to capture them reliably based on their expertise by defining adequate credible intervals (CrIs). The 5th, 50th and 95th percentiles (q_5, q_{50} and q_{95}) were chosen for CrI elicitation, as this is the most common practice in SEJs [56,65]. Through such 90% CrIs, participants express their beliefs that there is a 90% chance that the true mortality rate falls between q_5 and q_{95}.

2.9. Structured Expert Judgement Instruments

For each vignette, the following target question was posed: "According to you, what is the probability that a patient with these characteristics would die within 30 days after hip fracture surgery?" Participants were asked to choose a probability bin from the set (0–0.1), (0.1–0.2), . . ., (0.9–1.0), which reflected their beliefs best. The middle value of each bin functioned as a point estimate for pooling later in the analysis.

Calibration questions were based on 30-day mortality data from the Dutch Hip Fracture Audit Taskforce Indicators (DHFA-TFI) group [57], which described a total of 7506 patients. To ensure similarity with the target questions, calibration questions were based on patient subgroups, which resembled the vignettes. Similarity was ensured through age matching ($\geq$80 years) and choosing overlapping attributes: gender, fracture type, dementia, functional status in ADL, ASA scores and institutional residence. Since these characteristics were insufficient to construct ample diverse calibration questions, mobility, malnutrition and anaemia were included as additional attributes. An example of a calibration question is: "How many percent of the hip fracture patients aged **90 years or older**, who were **mobile without walking aids** and **did not have dementia**, died within 30 days following hip fracture surgery between 2017 and 2019, according to the DHFA-TFI group?" All 14 calibration questions can be found in Table A2 of Appendix A.

The ground truth of the calibration questions could not be obtained directly from the DHFA-TFI cohort since there were missing data. Information on 30-day mortality was missing for 19.5% of the 7506 patients. Missing entries were imputed with Multiple Imputation by Chained Equations (MICE) [58]. MICE was used to create 20 imputed data sets [58], from which the 30-day mortality percentages were extracted and pooled. With the true mortality rates available, participants' performances could be measured using two scoring metrics: the calibration score and the information score.

2.10. Expert Scoring and Performance Weighting

The calibration score evaluated the statistical accuracy of participants' CrIs. Calibration was measured by examining how well they captured the true 30-day mortality rates across the four inter-percentile ranges: $<q_5$, (q_5–q_{50}), (q_{50}–q_{95}) and $>q_{95}$. Participants were said to be well-calibrated if their 90% CrIs captured the true 30-day mortality rates across 90% of the calibration questions, such that the true values fell below q_5 in 5% of the cases, between q_5 and q_{50} in 45% of the cases, between q_{50} and q_{95} in 45% of the cases, and above q_{95} in 5% of the cases. The calibration score was defined as the p-value of a Chi-squared test examining whether the CrIs indeed captured the true mortality rates according to this theoretical distribution. A calibration score of 1 indicated the highest level of statistical accuracy.

The information score indicated the degree to which participants deemed some values more likely to be true than others. As they could in theory achieve perfect statistical accuracy by specifying overly wide CrIs, the information score was introduced to compensate for this. Participants received higher information scores if they specified more concentrated CrIs. The computational steps are described in more detail elsewhere [59].

Finally, the calibration scores and information scores were multiplied for each participant to obtain an overall performance weight. The weights were then normalised, such that they summed to 1 across all participants. For each vignette, the estimated probabilities of 30-day mortality were then combined into a performance-weighted average. Pooling with equal weights was performed as a sensitivity analysis.

3. Results

3.1. Respondents

In total, 21 survey responses were collected. These included 14 complete responses for the clinical vignette study (6 orthopaedic trauma surgeons and 8 surgical residents), of which 9 were also complete for the SEJ (4 orthopaedic trauma surgeons and 5 surgical residents). The medians and interquartile ranges of years of experience for orthopaedic trauma surgeons and surgical residents were 11.3 (8.5–18.1) and 4.0 (2.8–5.0), respectively.

3.2. Results of the Vignette Study

Table 3 depicts the outcomes of the vignette study. Amongst the inspected patient attributes, only four showcased 95% CrIs, which did not overlap with the null effect. In descending order of effect size, these were metastatic carcinoma (OR: 4.42, 95% CrI: 2.14–8.95), severe heart failure (OR: 4.05, 95% CrI: 1.89–8.29), end-stage renal failure (OR: 3.54, 95% CrI: 1.76–7.35) and dementia (OR: 3.35, 95% CrI: 1.70–7.06). From the estimated ORs, comorbid conditions appeared to affect the likelihood of recommending P-NOM the most. For instance, the odds that patients with metastatic carcinomas received a P-NOM recommendation were 4.42 times higher than for patients without metastatic carcinomas.

Table 3. Influence of patient characteristics on preferences for palliative non-operative management. Differences in odds ratios due to prior assumptions are quantified as relative deviations.

Attribute	Level	Informative Priors		Noninformative Priors		Deviation
		Odds Ratio	95% CrI	Odds Ratio	95% CrI	
Metastatic carcinoma	Present Absent *	4.42	**2.14–8.95**	6.41	**2.43–16.78**	45.0%
Severe heart failure	Present Absent *	4.05	**1.89–8.29**	4.72	**2.13–11.48**	16.5%
End-stage renal failure	Present Absent *	3.54	**1.76–7.35**	3.70	**1.56–8.86**	4.5%
Dementia	Present Absent *	3.35	**1.70–7.06**	3.96	**1.75–10.03**	18.2%
Physical status	ASA IV ASA III *	1.92	0.92–4.37	1.49	0.63–3.84	22.4%
Preoperative residence	Institution Home *	1.85	0.97–3.59	1.90	0.81–4.36	2.7%
Functional status	Severe handicaps No severe handicaps *	1.71	0.83–3.49	1.65	0.72–3.81	3.5%
Gender	Male Female *	1.55	0.74–3.42	1.53	0.67–3.58	1.3%
Age	≥90 years 80–89 years *	1.20	0.54–2.59	1.12	0.49–2.56	6.7%
Fracture type	Displaced femoral neck Extracapsular Undisplaced femoral neck *	1.00 0.81	0.41–2.41 0.34–1.92	0.85 0.67	0.32–2.34 0.26–1.83	15.0% 17.3%

* Reference level. The 95% CrIs displayed in bold are strictly non-overlapping with the null effect.

For all regression coefficients, the diagnostic tests indicated that the estimates were stable (see Appendix B). Furthermore, all substantive conclusions, that is, whether the CrIs were non-overlapping with the null effect, were robust with respect to the decreased informativeness of priors. The sensitivity analysis showed that the informative priors had little influence on the ORs of end-stage renal failure, preoperative residence, functional status, gender and age. The prior influence was moderate for severe heart failure, dementia and fracture type. Finally, priors were highly influential for the effect estimates of metastatic carcinoma and physical status.

3.3. Results of the Structured Expert Judgement

Figure 2 depicts the responses to the 14 calibration questions of nine participants who completed the SEJ. Only two participants (surgical residents) managed to achieve calibration scores above 0.05, indicating that they were well-calibrated. With calibration scores of 0.53 and 0.32, their judgements accounted for a cumulative normalised weight of 93% in the performance-weighted pooled estimates.

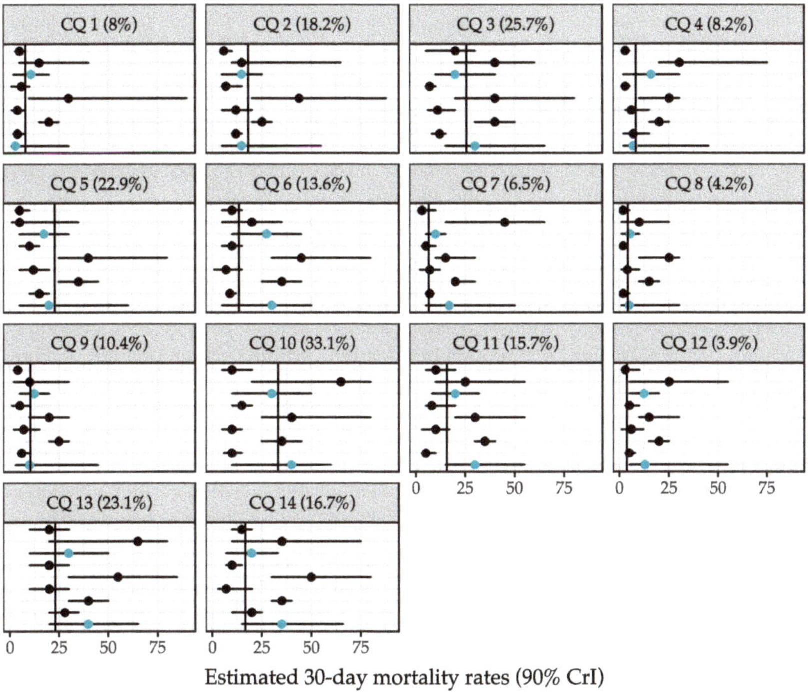

Figure 2. Overview of participants' responses to the 14 calibration questions. The dots represent participants' best estimates of the 30-day mortality rates and the horizontal bars represent their 90% credible intervals. The true 30-day mortality rate is reported in parentheses and depicted by the vertical line. Participants with calibration scores above 0.05 are highlighted in blue.

An overview of the 30-day mortality probability estimates obtained through linear opinion pooling with equal weights and performance-based weights is shown in Figure 3b. For each vignette, the performance-based weights estimates were consistently lower than the equal weights estimates. This entailed that those who had high calibration scores, estimated lower mortality risks than the average participants in the study sample. The pooled probabilities across all vignettes ranged between 20.7–62.7% and 11.9–50.8% for equal and performance-based weights, respectively.

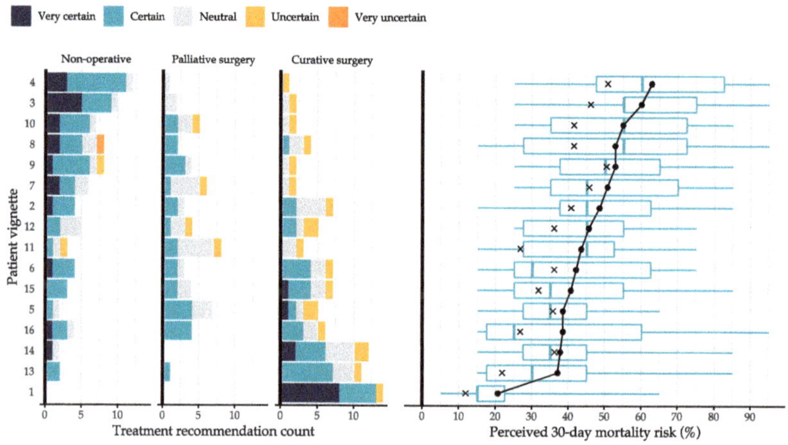

(a) (b)

Figure 3. Distribution of participants' responses to the 16 vignettes. Vignettes were sorted in descending order of mean 30-day mortality risk. (**a**) Overview of recommended treatments per vignette, subcategorised by participants' confidence in the optimality of the elected treatment. (**b**) Boxplots of the estimated 30-day mortality risks per vignette. Circles denote the mean probabilities (equal weights) and crosses denote the performance-weighted pooled estimates.

3.4. Heterogeneity in Treatment Preferences and Risk Perceptions

The trends shown in Figure 3 indicated that P-NOM was more frequently recommended to patients for whom a higher 30-day mortality risk was prognosticated on average. However, preferences for P-NOM differed considerably from participant to participant. The ICC was estimated at 0.299, which entailed that personal differences between participants explained 29.9% of the treatment recommendations. The apparent preference heterogeneity can be further exemplified by examining the P-NOM choice proportions across individual participants (see Table 4). On the highest extreme, four orthopaedic trauma surgeons each recommended P-NOM 10–12 times. On the lowest extreme, four surgical residents each recommended P-NOM 0–3 times. Hence, although participants expressed low degrees of uncertainty in the optimality of their elected treatments (see Figure 3a), their recommendations were divided.

Table 4. Summary of responses to the vignette study and structured expert judgement on participant level. Responses have been summarised across all 16 vignettes, with the risk range referring to the mortality risk for the best- and worst-case survival patients as estimated by the orthopaedic trauma surgeon/surgical resident.

Profession	Experience	P-NOM Recommendations	Risk Range
Orthopaedic trauma surgeon	>10 years	12/16 vignettes	35–95%
Orthopaedic trauma surgeon	>10 years	10/16 vignettes	25–65%
Orthopaedic trauma surgeon	>10 years	4/16 vignettes	35–75%
Orthopaedic trauma surgeon	5–10 years	12/16 vignettes	15–65%
Orthopaedic trauma surgeon	5–10 years	11/16 vignettes	5–35%
Orthopaedic trauma surgeon	5–10 years	3/16 vignettes	15–55%
Surgical resident	5–10 years	7/16 vignettes	15–85%
Surgical resident	5–10 years	3/16 vignettes	5–55%
Surgical resident	5–10 years	2/16 vignettes	5–65%
Surgical resident	<5 years	8/16 vignettes	15–55%
Surgical resident	<5 years	4/16 vignettes	15–95%
Surgical resident	<5 years	2/16 vignettes	65–95%
Surgical resident	<5 years	2/16 vignettes	15–75%
Surgical resident	<5 years	0/16 vignettes	15–35%

Furthermore, as shown in Figure 3b, participants' perceptions of 30-day mortality risks were also highly dispersed. For vignettes 8 and 16, for instance, the estimated prognoses varied between 15 and 95%. On the individual participant level, a difference in how sensitive their risk perceptions were to changes in patient attributes was observed as well (see Table 4). For three participants, the perceived mortality risk between the best- and worst-case survival patients only differed by 20–30 percentage points. For five others, this difference was 60–80 percentage points.

3.5. Participants' Feedback

In total, nine participants provided feedback on what information they missed in the vignette descriptions. Two participants expressed that they did not need any additional information. The remaining participants expressed a wish for more clinical details, that is, patients' pulmonary status, survival prognoses for metastatic cancer, mobility status, and the motivation behind high ASA scores. Additionally, participants expressed that aspects of real-life decision-making were lacking in the vignettes. For example, second opinions from geriatricians, anaesthesiologists and cardiologists could have helped in shaping a better treatment proposal. Furthermore, the nuances of being able to look patients in the eye and ask them and their relatives about their personal treatment preferences were deemed important in real-life decision-making as well.

4. Discussion

This paper reports on the first quantitative decision analysis of surgical residents' and orthopaedic trauma surgeons' P-NOM recommendations for hypothetical cases of frail geriatric hip fracture patients. The results showed that metastatic carcinoma, severe heart failure, end-stage renal failure and dementia had the strongest influence on their preferences to recommend P-NOM. While cancer, renal insufficiency and dementia were already identified as common comorbidities in non-operatively treated hip fracture patients [13], we are the first to quantify their impact on physicians' treatment recommendations. Furthermore, we found that preferences for P-NOM generally increased with perceived mortality risks. These findings underline and confirm that comorbidities leading to increased mortality risk are some of the strongest indicators to favour P-NOM over surgery [8,66].

However, some of these findings were unexpected, given the a priori hypotheses. First, based on the power analysis with an assumed OR of 1.4, no significant effect was expected to be found for the influence of dementia. In fact, with an observed OR of 3.35, dementia appeared to have a substantially higher influence on preferences for P-NOM than hypothesised. Second, the estimated effect size of metastatic carcinoma appeared to be highly influenced by the specification of the informative prior. The a priori assumed OR of 2.5 was substantially smaller than the observed ORs of 4.42 (2.14–8.95) and 6.41 (2.43–16.78) for informative and noninformative priors, respectively. This gives rise to the question of whether the influence of these attributes was undervalued in the a priori hypotheses or whether participants overvalued these attributes.

In retrospect, we would like to plead for the former. The a priori assumed effect sizes of the attributes were solely estimated based on their prognostic value for 30-day mortality. Initially, the assumption was made that 30-mortality risk could function as a viable proxy to model the ORs in the vignette study, since the risk of early death is a leading argument to elect P-NOM according to the national guidelines [8]. However, 30-day mortality risk alone may not be sufficient to fully encompass the benefit of P-NOM, as it overlooks QoL considerations [9]. A previous study found that over 90% of the 271 surveyed healthcare providers expressed that a poor postoperative QoL prospect was a common reason for them to treat frail geriatric hip fracture patients non-operatively [66]. Hence, we may have undervalued the influence of dementia and metastatic carcinomas in the priors as QoL was not accounted for. To substantiate these claims, important QoL considerations for both conditions will be delineated.

First, it is increasingly acknowledged that dementia is a terminal condition [67–69] that necessitates palliative care assessments [70]. This necessity is particularly pronounced in the advanced stages of dementia, with inclinations towards self-neglect in the form of malnutrition due to dysphagia [67]. In end-of-life care for demented older adults, Dutch clinicians agree that forgoing artificial nutrition and hydration (ANH) could be good medical practice [71], as ANH prolongs patients' lives at the expense of serious discomfort [72]. Hence, safeguarding the QoL of demented patients may in fact entail safeguarding a humane death. However, these circumstances may not be applicable to all demented hip fracture patients, but primarily to those with advanced dementia [18]. Nevertheless, since preoperative dementia is a well-known significant risk factor for postoperative delirium, surgery may accelerate patients' cognitive decline [42–44]. With these outcomes in mind, the perceived benefit of P-NOM may come from poor postoperative QoL prognoses, on top of increased mortality risk.

Second, recovery-oriented surgery is unlikely to improve the well-being of geriatric hip fracture patients who are debilitated by advanced malignancy [6]. While pain reduction could be a viable reason to elect surgery [73], the treatment's benefit depends on the patient's age and health status. Preference studies have shown that cancer patients aged 65 years and older are less willing to trade prolonged survival for decreased QoL than their younger counterparts [74]. Especially for those who are frail and suffer from metastasis, the best supportive care could be preferred due to its acceptable outcomes with respect to QoL [75–77]. Therefore, considering the implications of frailty and patients' end-of-life preferences, QoL aspects may have contributed to the perceived benefit of P-NOM for hip fracture patients with metastatic cancer.

While several patient attributes were found to be critical for preoperative decision-making, it should be noted that treatment preferences were rather heterogeneous. On the one hand, heterogeneity in stated preferences could be attributable to the simplified nature of the vignettes, leading to a lack of nuances, which could have helped participants assess the patient cases more confidently and reliably. On the other hand, even for vignettes where participants consistently expressed (high) certainty for the optimality of their treatment recommendations, stated preferences remained divided. These observations are most likely reflecting the lack of guidelines for considering P-NOM.

Besides that, substantial heterogeneity in 30-day mortality risk perceptions was observed as well. This exemplifies the need for objective 30-day mortality prediction models to streamline risk perceptions. Through the SEJ, an attempt was made to forge a rational consensus between participants' dispersed risk estimates. Through linear opinion pooling with performance-based weights, the expert judgements yielded a 30-day mortality prediction range between 11.9 and 50.8% across all vignettes. However, the maximum risk estimate appeared to be rather low, considering that it was the prognosis for a male institutionalised ASA IV patient between the ages of 80 and 89 years with severe functional handicaps, severe heart failure, metastatic cancer and end-stage renal failure.

To place the expert-driven estimates into perspective, a comparison was made with data-driven prediction models. An overview of the maximum predicted risks and the respective predictor variables of the Nottingham Hip Fracture Score (NHFS) [22], Almelo Hip Fracture Score (AHFS) [20], $AHFS^{90}$ [78] and Brabant Hip Fracture Score (BHFS) [21] is shown in Table 5. This overview shows that most predictors also appear in the vignettes. The vignettes, however, include three strong predictors for 30-day mortality that are not included in the prediction models: metastatic cancer, severe heart failure and end-stage renal failure. Based on our systematic review [35], we observed that these predictors have larger effect sizes than most of the other predictors considered in the NHFS, AHFS, $AHFS^{90}$ and BHFS. Yet, the performance-based weights estimate only attained a marginally higher maximum risk than the NHFS and BHFS. In comparison to the AHFS and the $AHFS^{90}$, physicians' collective judgements were lower, regardless of using equal or performance-based weights. As the maximum AHFS and $AHFS^{90}$ were computed in a relatively healthy population compared to the vignettes, physicians' collective estimates are likely downward biassed for the most vulnerable patients. Thus, patients at high risk of early mortality are potentially underidentified in practice.

Table 5. Comparison of maximum 30-day mortality risks as estimated by prediction models and physicians' judgements. Attributes included in prediction models/vignette are marked with an X.

Attribute	30-Day Mortality Prediction Models				Physicians	
	NHFS (45.0%)	AHFS (68.4%)	AHFS^{90} (64.5%)	BHFS (46.6%)	EW (62.9%)	PW (50.8%)
Age	X	X	X	X	X	X
Gender	X	X	X	X	X	X
Preoperative residence	X	X	X	X	X	X
History of malignancy	X	X		X	X [1]	X [1]
Cognitive impairment	X	X	X		X	X
Admission haemoglobin	X	X	X	X		
ASA classification		X	X		X	X
Number of comorbidities	X	X				
Mobility		X				
COPD				X		
Diabetes				X		
Functional status					X	X
Severe heart failure					X	X
End-stage renal failure					X	X
Fracture type					X	X

NHFS Nottingham Hip Fracture Score, AHFS Almelo Hip Fracture Score, AHFS^{90} Almelo Hip Fracture Score in patients aged ≥90 years, BHFS Brabant Hip Fracture Score, EW equally weighted pooled estimate, PW performance-weighted pooled estimate, ASA American Society of Anesthesiologists physical status classification, COPD chronic obstructive pulmonary disease. [1] Malignancy was exclusively defined as metastatic cancer.

However, several limitations may have downward biassed the equal and performance-based weight estimates for the most vulnerable patients. Since only nine participants completed the SEJ, underestimations may have been observed due to chance. Replication of the study in a larger cohort is necessary to confirm the findings. Nevertheless, two well-calibrated surgical residents were observed in this sample, accounting for a cumulative weight of 93% in the pooled estimates. Based on the premise of the SEJ, it is counterintuitive that they underestimated the 30-day mortality risk for the most vulnerable patients. It is postulated that the calibration questions did not capture the relevant range of expertise for the diverse vignettes, as the questions' true realisations were limited to 30-day mortality rates between 3.9 and 33.2%. As the SEJ instrument calibrated participants to relatively healthy patients, a high calibration score did not reflect accurate predictions for high-risk patients. Future researchers should examine how the limited data on high-risk patients can be used more effectively to develop representative calibration questions.

Another limitation of this study was that the multi-faceted decision context was solely represented by surgical residents and orthopaedic trauma surgeons. Recommending adequate palliative care remains a challenging task, as trade-offs are to be made between relieving pain through surgery with risks of iatrogenesis [10,11] and resorting to analgesics in P-NOM with higher risks of pain undertreatment [9]. In our study, the participants expressed that the perspectives of other clinicians, such as geriatricians and anaesthesiologists, could have helped in improving the adequacy of the treatment proposals. Affirmatively, studies have shown that consultations with geriatricians were highly influential in the preoperative decision-making process [18]. Hence, the expertise from a broader group of clinical stakeholders may be necessary to adequately develop guidelines for considering P-NOM.

Finally, the results of the vignette study should be interpreted with caution due to the small sample size. According to our a priori power analysis, the study was only sufficiently powered for a few attributes: metastatic carcinoma, severe heart failure and end-stage renal failure. Increasing the sample size will likely result in the detection of meaningful effects for physical status, preoperative residence and functional status, since the ORs of these attributes have 95% CrIs, which are close to non-overlapping with the null effect. As it may be challenging to enrol sufficient participants, our posterior distributions could be used as highly informative priors in future work. By systematically updating the evidence found in this study through a Bayesian framework, the foundations laid here may strongly alleviate large sample size requirements in future studies.

5. Conclusions

This study demonstrated that the presence of metastatic carcinomas (OR: 4.42, CrI: 2.14–8.95), severe heart failure (OR: 4.05, CrI: 1.89–8.29), end-stage renal failure (OR: 3.54, CrI: 1.76–7.35) and dementia (OR: 3.35, CrI: 1.70–7.06) had the strongest influence on the decisions of surgical residents and orthopaedic trauma surgeons to favour P-NOM in frail geriatric hip fracture patients. Although they were more inclined to abstain from surgery amongst patients for whom higher 30-day mortality risks were prognosticated on average, heterogeneity in treatment preferences and risk perceptions was substantial. Hence, objective 30-day mortality prediction models should be used in clinical practice to streamline risk perceptions. However, objective mortality risk estimates alone are postulated to be insufficient to identify eligible candidates for P-NOM. Although meta-analyses revealed that some of the examined attributes were of small-to-moderate prognostic value for 30-day mortality, surgical residents and orthopaedic trauma surgeons could still strongly associate them with favouring P-NOM. The increased impact of these attributes is presumably derived from poor postoperative QoL prognoses, in addition to increased 30-day mortality risk. Hence, based on the stated preferences, more emphasis may need to be put on QoL considerations in clinical guidelines, to adequately provide decision support for considering P-NOM.

Author Contributions: Conceptualisation, M.B., C.G.M.G.-O., A.W. and J.H.H.; methodology, M.B., C.G.M.G.-O., A.W. and J.H.H.; software, M.B. and C.G.M.G.-O.; validation, M.B.; formal analysis, M.B.; investigation, M.B. and J.H.H.; resources, M.B. and J.H.H.; data curation, M.B.; writing—original draft preparation, M.B.; writing—review and editing, M.B., C.G.M.G.-O., A.W. and J.H.H.; visualisation, M.B.; supervision, C.G.M.G.-O., A.W. and J.H.H.; project administration, M.B. All authors have read and agreed to the published version of the manuscript.

Funding: This research received no external funding.

Institutional Review Board Statement: The study was exempt from the Medical Research Involving Human Subjects Act and approved by the ethical committee of Computer & Information Science of the University of Twente (protocol code: RP 2022-118 and date of approval: 14-06-2022).

Informed Consent Statement: Informed consent was obtained from all subjects involved in the study.

Data Availability Statement: The data are not available as no consent was obtained from the participants to share the raw data.

Acknowledgments: The authors would like to thank G.F. Nane for her advice on the structured expert judgement methodology.

Conflicts of Interest: The authors declare no conflicts of interest.

Appendix A

Table A1. Complete descriptions of the 16 vignettes included in the experimental design.

ID	ASA	Fracture	Gender	Age	Severe Functional Handicaps	Residence	Dementia	Severe Heart Failure	Metastasis	ESRF
1	III	DFN	Female	80–89	No	Home	No	No	No	No
2	IV	UFN	Female	90+	No	Home	No	Yes	No	Yes
3	IV	DFN	Female	90+	No	Institution	Yes	No	Yes	Yes
4	IV	EXT	Male	80–89	Yes	Institution	No	Yes	Yes	Yes
5	IV	EXT	Female	90+	Yes	Home	No	No	Yes	No
6	III	DFN	Male	80–89	Yes	Home	Yes	No	No	Yes
7	IV	UFN	Female	80–89	Yes	Institution	Yes	No	No	Yes

Table A1. *Cont.*

ID	ASA	Fracture	Gender	Age	Severe Functional Handicaps	Residence	Dementia	Severe Heart Failure	Metastasis	ESRF
8	IV	UFN	Male	80–89	No	Home	Yes	Yes	Yes	No
9	IV	DFN	Male	90+	Yes	Home	Yes	Yes	Yes	No
10	III	EXT	Female	90+	Yes	Home	Yes	Yes	Yes	Yes
11	IV	DFN	Female	80–89	Yes	Institution	No	Yes	Yes	No
12	III	DFN	Male	90+	No	Institution	No	Yes	Yes	Yes
13	III	UFN	Male	90+	Yes	Institution	No	No	Yes	No
14	IV	EXT	Male	80–89	No	Home	No	No	Yes	Yes
15	IV	EXT	Male	90+	No	Institution	Yes	No	Yes	No
16	III	EXT	Female	80–89	No	Institution	Yes	Yes	Yes	No

ASA American Society of Anesthesiologists physical status classification, ESRF end-stage renal failure, DFN displaced femoral neck, UFN undisplaced femoral neck, EXT extracapsular.

Table A2. Overview of calibration questions and the corresponding 30-day mortality rates according to the Dutch Hip Fracture Audit Taskforce Indicators (DHFA-TF) group.

ID	Calibration Question	Mortality
1	How many percent of the **female** hip fracture patients aged **80 years or older** died within 30 days following hip fracture surgery between 2017 and 2019, according to the DHFA-TFI group?	8.0%
2	How many percent of the **male** hip fracture patients aged **90 years or older** died within 30 days following hip fracture surgery between 2017 and 2019, according to the DHFA-TFI group?	18.3%
3	How many percent of the hip fracture patients aged **85 years or older** with an **ASA IV classification** died within 30 days following hip fracture surgery between 2017 and 2019, according to the DHFA-TFI group?	25.9%
4	How many percent of the hip fracture patients aged **80 years or older** with an **ASA II-III classification** died within 30 days following hip fracture surgery between 2017 and 2019, according to the DHFA-TFI group?	8.2%
5	How many percent of the hip fracture patients aged **80 years or older** with a **high risk of malnutrition** (SNAQ score $\geq$ 3) and **pre-fracture institutional residence** died within 30 days following hip fracture surgery between 2017 and 2019, according to the DHFA-TFI group?	22.8%
6	How many percent of the hip fracture patients aged **80 years or older** with a **high risk of malnutrition** (SNAQ score $\geq$ 3) and **preoperative anaemia** died within 30 days following hip fracture surgery between 2017 and 2019, according to the DHFA-TFI group?	13.9%
7	How many percent of the hip fracture patients aged **80 years or older** with a **displaced femoral neck fracture** died within 30 days following hip fracture surgery between 2017 and 2019, according to the DHFA-TFI group?	6.5%
8	How many percent of the hip fracture patients aged **80 years or older** who were **fully independent in activities of daily living** (Katz score of 6) and at **low risk of malnutrition** (SNAQ score $\geq$ 1) died within 30 days following hip fracture surgery between 2017 and 2019, according to the DHFA-TFI group?	4.2%
9	How many percent of the hip fracture patients aged **90 years or older**, who were **mobile without walking aids** and **did not have dementia**, died within 30 days following hip fracture surgery between 2017 and 2019, according to the DHFA-TFI group?	10.2%
10	How many percent of the hip fracture patients aged **80 years or older** with an **ASA IV classification** and **prefracture institutional residence** died within 30 days following hip fracture surgery between 2017 and 2019, according to the DHFA-TFI group?	33.2%
11	How many percent of the hip fracture patients aged **90 years or older** with an **extracapsular fracture** and **preoperative anaemia** died within 30 days following hip fracture surgery between 2017 and 2019, according to the DHFA-TFI group?	15.7%
12	How many percent of the hip fracture patients aged **90 years or older** with an **ASA I-II classification** died within 30 days following hip fracture surgery between 2017 and 2019, according to the DHFA-TFI group?	3.9%
13	How many percent of the hip fracture patients aged **90 years or older** with an **ASA III-IV** classification, dementia and **pre-fracture institutional residence** died within 30 days following hip fracture surgery between 2017 and 2019, according to the DHFA-TFI group?	23.2%
14	How many percent of the hip fracture patients aged **90 years or older** with **severe functional handicaps** (Katz score 0–2) died within 30 days following hip fracture surgery between 2017 and 2019, according to the DHFA-TFI group?	16.7%

Katz and SNAQ scores were explained to the participants. Patient characteristics of interest were emphasised in bold to improve the readability of the calibration questions in the survey.

Appendix B

Convergence of the Markov chains was confirmed visually by inspection of the trace plots (see Figures A1–A3) and autocorrelation plots (see Figure A4). The trendless trace plots and rapid decays in the autocorrelation plots were indicative of healthy convergence. Furthermore, Geweke's convergence test yielded p-values above 0.05 for all regression coefficients, implying that stationarity could be assumed. Upon inspecting the frequency histograms of the posterior draws (see Figure A5), the distributions appeared to be smooth without substantial gaps between the bins. Hence, 15,000 samples were ample enough to adequately represent the posterior distributions.

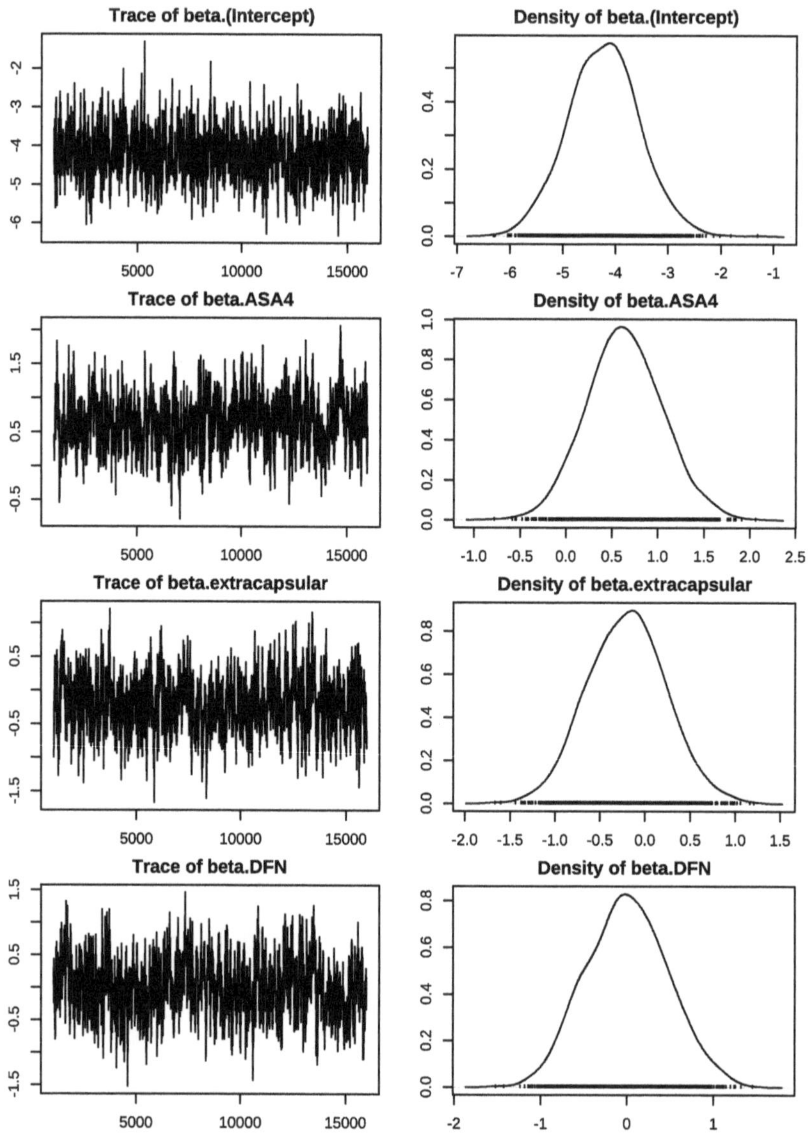

Figure A1. Trace plots and densities of the posterior distributions of the coefficients (1/3).

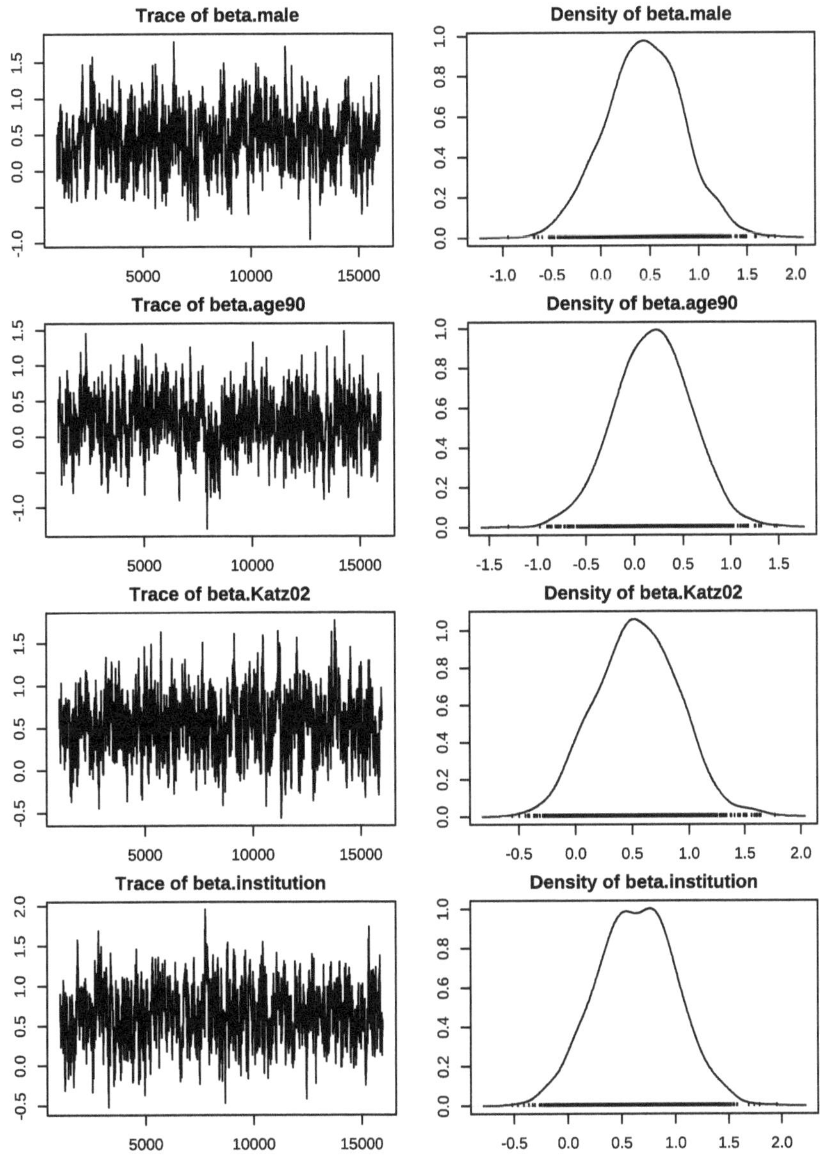

Figure A2. Trace plots and densities of the posterior distributions of the coefficients (2/3).

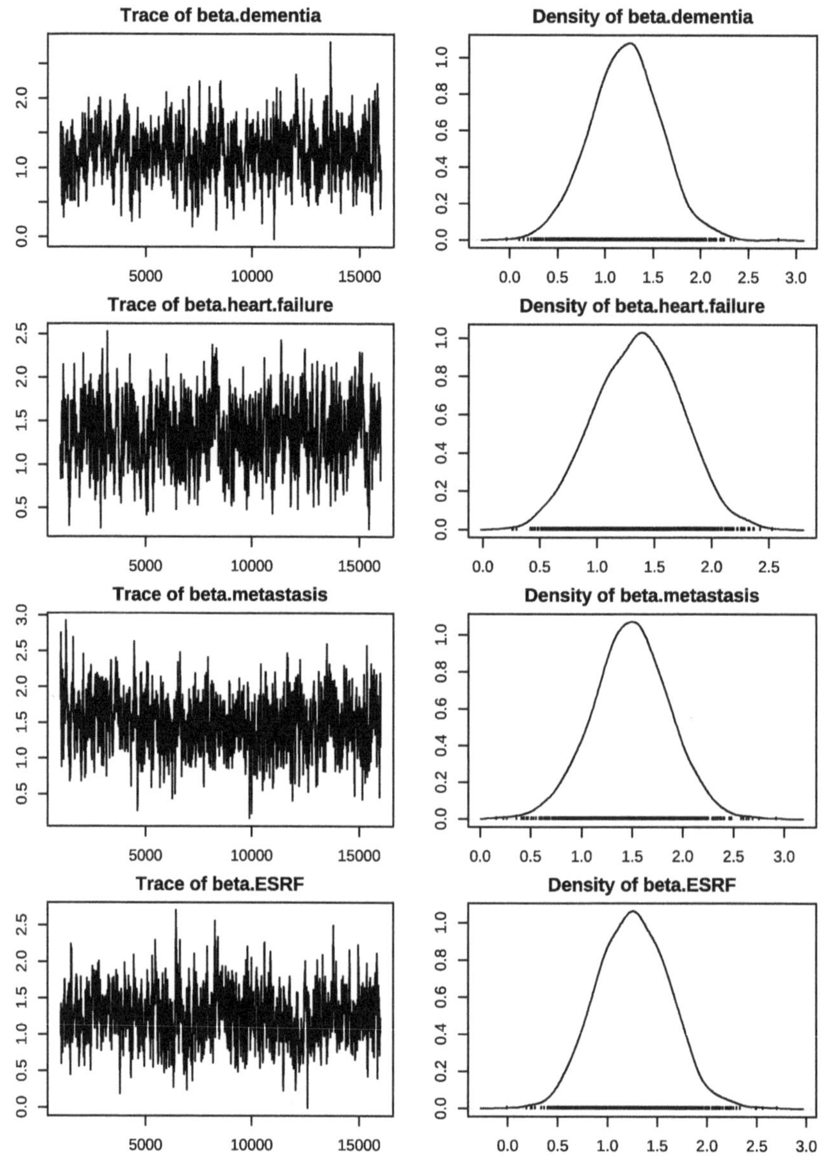

Figure A3. Trace plots and densities of the posterior distributions of the coefficients (3/3).

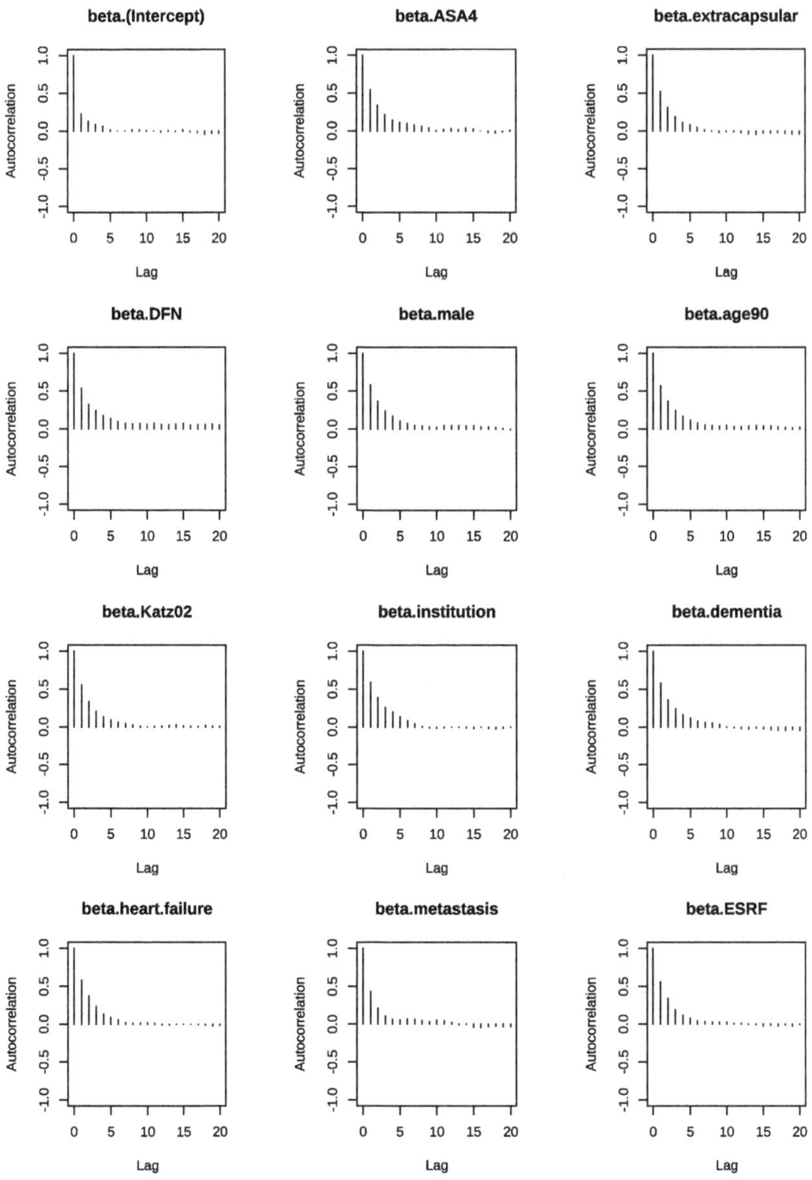

Figure A4. Autocorrelation plots of the Markov chains for each regression coefficient.

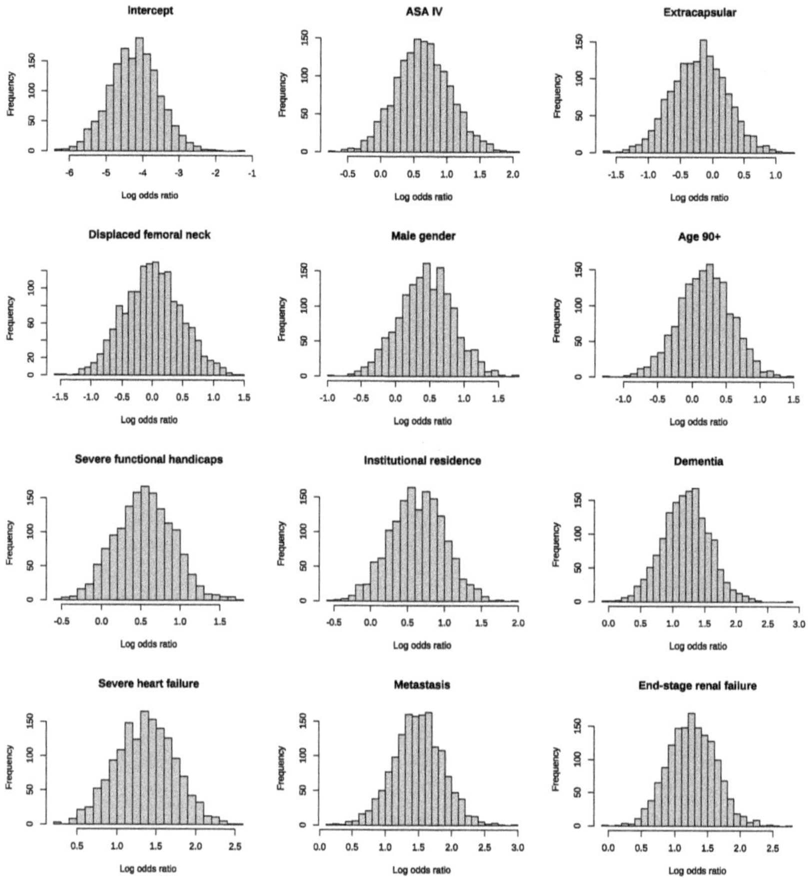

Figure A5. Histograms of the posterior samples drawn through Markov Chain Monte Carlo sampling for each regression coefficient.

References

1. Bhandari, M.; Swiontkowski, M. Management of Acute Hip Fracture. *N. Engl. J. Med.* **2017**, *377*, 2053–2062. [CrossRef]
2. Parker, M.; Johansen, A. Hip Fracture. *BMJ* **2006**, *333*, 27–30. [CrossRef] [PubMed]
3. van de Ree, C.L.P.; De Jongh, M.A.C.; Peeters, C.M.M.; de Munter, L.; Roukema, J.A.; Gosens, T. Hip Fractures in Elderly People Surgery or No Surgery? A Systematic Review and Meta-Analysis. *Geriatr. Orthop. Surg. Rehabil.* **2017**, *8*, 173–180. [CrossRef] [PubMed]
4. Kim, S.-J.; Park, H.-S.; Lee, D.-W. Outcome of Nonoperative Treatment for Hip Fractures in Elderly Patients: A Systematic Review of Recent Literature. *J. Orthop. Surg.* **2020**, *28*, 2309499020936848. [CrossRef]
5. Berry, S.D.; Rothbaum, R.R.; Kiel, D.P.; Lee, Y.; Mitchell, S.L. Association of Clinical Outcomes with Surgical Repair of Hip Fracture vs Nonsurgical Management in Nursing Home Residents with Advanced Dementia. *JAMA Intern. Med.* **2018**, *178* 774–780. [CrossRef] [PubMed]
6. McNamara, P.; Sharma, K. Surgery or Palliation for Hip Fractures in Patients with Advanced Malignancy? *Age Ageing* **1997**, *26* 471–474. [CrossRef] [PubMed]
7. Cannada, L.K.; Mears, S.C.; Quatman, C. Clinical Faceoff: When Should Patients 65 Years of Age and Older Have Surgery for Hip Fractures, and When Is It a Bad Idea? *Clin. Orthop. Relat. Res.* **2021**, *479*, 24–27. [CrossRef] [PubMed]
8. Federatie Medisch Specialisten Richtlijn Proximale Femurfracturen. Available online: https://richtlijnendatabase.nl/richtlijn/behandeling_kwetsbare_ouderen_bij_chirurgie/proximale_femurfractuur_preoperatieve_traject/besluitvorming_bij_proximale_femurfractuur.html (accessed on 20 April 2022).

9. Loggers, S.A.I.; Willems, H.C.; Van Balen, R.; Gosens, T.; Polinder, S.; Ponsen, K.J.; Van de Ree, C.L.P.; Steens, J.; Verhofstad, M.H.J.; Zuurmond, R.G.; et al. Evaluation of Quality of Life after Nonoperative or Operative Management of Proximal Femoral Fractures in Frail Institutionalized Patients: The FRAIL-HIP Study. *JAMA Surg.* **2022**, *157*, 424–434. [CrossRef]
10. Clapp, J.T.; Schwarze, M.L.; Fleisher, L.A. Surgical Overtreatment and Shared Decision-Making—The Limits of Choice. *JAMA Surg.* **2022**, *157*, 5–6. [CrossRef]
11. Cardona-Morrell, M.; Kim, J.; Turner, R.M.; Anstey, M.; Mitchell, I.A.; Hillman, K. Non-Beneficial Treatments in Hospital at the End of Life: A Systematic Review on Extent of the Problem. *Int. J. Qual. Health Care* **2016**, *28*, 456–469. [CrossRef]
12. Nijdam, T.M.P.; Laane, D.W.P.M.; Spierings, J.F.; Schuijt, H.J.; Smeeing, D.P.J.; van der Velde, D. Proxy-Reported Experiences of Palliative, Non-Operative Management of Geriatric Patients after a Hip Fracture: A Qualitative Study. *BMJ Open* **2022**, *12*, e063007. [CrossRef]
13. Loggers, S.A.I.; Van Lieshout, E.M.M.; Joosse, P.; Verhofstad, M.H.J.; Willems, H.C. Prognosis of Nonoperative Treatment in Elderly Patients with a Hip Fracture: A Systematic Review and Meta-Analysis. *Injury* **2020**, *51*, 2407–2413. [CrossRef]
14. Wijnen, H.H.; Schmitz, P.P.; Es-Safraouy, H.; Roovers, L.A.; Taekema, D.G.; Van Susante, J.L.C. Nonoperative Management of Hip Fractures in Very Frail Elderly Patients May Lead to a Predictable Short Survival as Part of Advance Care Planning. *Acta Orthop.* **2021**, *92*, 728–732. [CrossRef]
15. Ko, F.C.; Morrison, R.S. Hip Fracture: A Trigger for Palliative Care in Vulnerable Older Adults. *JAMA Intern. Med.* **2014**, *174*, 1281–1282. [CrossRef]
16. Neuman, M.D.; Silber, J.H.; Magaziner, J.S.; Passarella, M.A.; Mehta, S.; Werner, R.M. Survival and Functional Outcomes after Hip Fracture among Nursing Home Residents. *JAMA Intern. Med.* **2014**, *174*, 1273–1280. [CrossRef] [PubMed]
17. Joosten, E.a.G.; DeFuentes-Merillas, L.; de Weert, G.H.; Sensky, T.; van der Staak, C.P.F.; Jong, C.A.J. de Systematic Review of the Effects of Shared Decision-Making on Patient Satisfaction, Treatment Adherence and Health Status. *Psychother. Psychosom.* **2008**, *77*, 219–226. [CrossRef] [PubMed]
18. van der Zwaard, B.C.; Stein, C.E.; Bootsma, J.E.M.; van Geffen, H.J.A.A.; Douw, C.M.; Keijsers, C.J.P.W. Fewer Patients Undergo Surgery When Adding a Comprehensive Geriatric Assessment in Older Patients with a Hip Fracture. *Arch. Orthop. Trauma. Surg.* **2020**, *140*, 487–492. [CrossRef]
19. Prommik, P.; Tootsi, K.; Saluse, T.; Märtson, A.; Kolk, H. Nonoperative Hip Fracture Management Practices and Patient Survival Compared to Surgical Care: An Analysis of Estonian Population-Wide Data. *Arch. Osteoporos.* **2021**, *16*, 101. [CrossRef]
20. Nijmeijer, W.S.; Folbert, E.C.; Vermeer, M.; Slaets, J.P.; Hegeman, J.H. Prediction of Early Mortality Following Hip Fracture Surgery in Frail Elderly: The Almelo Hip Fracture Score (AHFS). *Injury* **2016**, *47*, 2138–2143. [CrossRef] [PubMed]
21. van de Ree, C.L.; Gosens, T.; van der Veen, A.H.; Oosterbos, C.J.; Heymans, M.W.; de Jongh, M.A. Development and Validation of the Brabant Hip Fracture Score for 30-Day and 1-Year Mortality. *HIP Int.* **2020**, *30*, 354–362. [CrossRef] [PubMed]
22. Moppett, I.K.; Parker, M.; Griffiths, R.; Bowers, T.; White, S.M.; Moran, C.G. Nottingham Hip Fracture Score: Longitudinal and Multi-Centre Assessment. *Br. J. Anaesth.* **2012**, *109*, 546–550. [CrossRef]
23. Yenidogan, B.; Pathak, S.; Geerdink, J.; Hegeman, J.H.; van Keulen, M. Multimodal Machine Learning for 30-Days Post-Operative Mortality Prediction of Elderly Hip Fracture Patients. In Proceedings of the 2021 International Conference on Data Mining Workshops (ICDMW), Auckland, New Zealand, 7–10 December 2021; pp. 508–516.
24. Cary, M.P.; Zhuang, F.; Draelos, R.L.; Pan, W.; Amarasekara, S.; Douthit, B.J.; Kang, Y.; Colón-Emeric, C.S. Machine Learning Algorithms to Predict Mortality and Allocate Palliative Care for Older Patients with Hip Fracture. *J. Am. Med. Dir. Assoc.* **2021**, *22*, 291–296. [CrossRef]
25. French, S.; Hanea, A.M.; Bedford, T.; Nane, G.F. Introduction and Overview of Structured Expert Judgement. In *Expert Judgement in Risk and Decision Analysis*; Hanea, A.M., Ed.; International Series in Operations Research and Management Science; Springer Open: Berlin/Heidelberg, Germany, 2021; pp. 1–16.
26. Hanea, A.M.; Nane, G.F. Calibrating Experts' Probabilistic Assessments for Improved Probabilistic Predictions. *Saf. Sci.* **2019**, *118*, 763–771. [CrossRef]
27. Quinn, R.H.; Mooar, P.A.; Murray, J.N.; Pezold, R.; Sevarino, K.S. Treatment of Hip Fractures in the Elderly. *J. Am. Acad. Orthop. Surg.* **2017**, *25*, e102–e104. [CrossRef]
28. Ryan, M.; Farrar, S. Using Conjoint Analysis to Elicit Preferences for Health Care. *BMJ* **2000**, *320*, 1530–1533. [CrossRef] [PubMed]
29. Ryan, M.; Scott, D.A.; Reeves, C.; Bate, A.; van Teijlingen, E.R.; Russell, E.M.; Napper, M.; Robb, C.M. Eliciting Public Preferences for Healthcare: A Systematic Review of Techniques. *Health Technol. Assess.* **2001**, *5*, 25–39. [CrossRef] [PubMed]
30. Bachmann, L.M.; Mühleisen, A.; Bock, A.; ter Riet, G.; Held, U.; Kessels, A.G. Vignette Studies of Medical Choice and Judgement to Study Caregivers' Medical Decision Behaviour: Systematic Review. *BMC Med. Res. Methodol.* **2008**, *8*, 50. [CrossRef] [PubMed]
31. Atzmüller, C.; Steiner, P.M. Experimental Vignette Studies in Survey Research. *Methodology* **2010**, *6*, 128–138. [CrossRef]
32. Evans, S.C.; Roberts, M.C.; Keeley, J.W.; Blossom, J.B.; Amaro, C.M.; Garcia, A.M.; Stough, C.O.; Canter, K.S.; Robles, R.; Reed, G.M. Vignette Methodologies for Studying Clinicians' Decision-Making: Validity, Utility, and Application in ICD-11 Field Studies. *Int. J. Clin. Health Psychol.* **2015**, *15*, 160–170. [CrossRef]
33. Taylor, B.J. Factorial Surveys: Using Vignettes to Study Professional Judgement. *Br. J. Soc. Work* **2006**, *36*, 1187–1207. [CrossRef]
34. Cooke, R.M. *Experts in Uncertainty: Opinion and Subjective Probability in Science*; Oxford University Press: Oxford, UK, 1991; ISBN 0-19-506465-8.

35. Bui, M.; Nijmeijer, W.S.; Hegeman, J.H.; Witteveen, A.; Groothuis-Oudshoorn, C.G.M. Systematic Review and Meta-Analysis of Preoperative Predictors for Early Mortality Following Hip Fracture Surgery. *Osteoporos. Int.* **2023**. [CrossRef]
36. Daabiss, M. American Society of Anaesthesiologists Physical Status Classification. *Indian J. Anaesth.* **2011**, *55*, 111–115. [CrossRef] [PubMed]
37. de Groot, R.; Nijmeijer, W.S.; Folbert, E.C.; Vollenbroek-Hutten, M.M.R.; Hegeman, J.H. 'Nonagenarians' with a Hip Fracture: Is a Different Orthogeriatric Treatment Strategy Necessary? *Arch. Osteoporos.* **2020**, *15*, 19. [CrossRef] [PubMed]
38. Hurwitz, E.E.; Simon, M.; Vinta, S.R.; Zehm, C.F.; Shabot, S.M.; Minhajuddin, A.; Abouleish, A.E. Adding Examples to the ASA-Physical Status Classification Improves Correct Assignment to Patients. *Anesthesiology* **2017**, *126*, 614–622. [CrossRef] [PubMed]
39. Mayhew, D.; Mendonca, V.; Murthy, B.V.S. A Review of ASA Physical Status—Historical Perspectives and Modern Developments. *Anaesthesia* **2019**, *74*, 373–379. [CrossRef]
40. Sweitzer, N.K.; Lopatin, M.; Yancy, C.W.; Mills, R.M.; Stevenson, L.W. Comparison of Clinical Features and Outcomes of Patients Hospitalized with Heart Failure and Normal Ejection Fraction (> or =55%) versus Those with Mildly Reduced (40% to 55%) and Moderately to Severely Reduced (<40%) Fractions. *Am. J. Cardiol.* **2008**, *101*, 1151–1156. [CrossRef]
41. Stevens, L.A.; Viswanathan, G.; Weiner, D.E. Chronic Kidney Disease and End-Stage Renal Disease in the Elderly Population: Current Prevalence, Future Projections, and Clinical Significance. *Adv. Chronic Kidney Dis.* **2010**, *17*, 293–301. [CrossRef]
42. Smith, T.O.; Cooper, A.; Peryer, G.; Griffiths, R.; Fox, C.; Cross, J. Factors Predicting Incidence of Post-Operative Delirium in Older People Following Hip Fracture Surgery: A Systematic Review and Meta-Analysis. *Int. J. Geriatr. Psychiatry* **2017**, *32*, 386–396. [CrossRef]
43. Bitsch, M.; Foss, N.; Kristensen, B.; Kehlet, H. Pathogenesis of and Management Strategies for Postoperative Delirium after Hip fractureA Review. *Acta Orthop. Scand.* **2004**, *75*, 378–389. [CrossRef]
44. Mosk, C.A.; Mus, M.; Vroemen, J.P.; van der Ploeg, T.; Vos, D.I.; Elmans, L.H.; van der Laan, L. Dementia and Delirium, the Outcomes in Elderly Hip Fracture Patients. *Clin. Interv. Aging* **2017**, *12*, 421–430. [CrossRef]
45. Araujo, B.L.d.C.; Theobald, D. Letter to the Editor: ASA Physical Status Classification in Surgical Oncology and the Importance of Improving Inter-Rater Reliability. *J. Korean Med. Sci.* **2017**, *32*, 1211–1212. [CrossRef]
46. Johnson, F.R.; Lancsar, E.; Marshall, D.; Kilambi, V.; Mühlbacher, A.; Regier, D.A.; Bresnahan, B.W.; Kanninen, B.; Bridges, J.F.P. Constructing Experimental Designs for Discrete-Choice Experiments: Report of the ISPOR Conjoint Analysis Experimental Design Good Research Practices Task Force. *Value Health* **2013**, *16*, 3–13. [CrossRef]
47. de Aguiar, P.F.; Bourguignon, B.; Khots, M.S.; Massart, D.L.; Phan-Than-Luu, R. D-Optimal Designs. *Chemom. Intell. Lab. Syst.* **1995**, *30*, 199–210. [CrossRef]
48. Morgan-Wall, T.; Khoury, G. Optimal Design Generation and Power Evaluation in R: The Skpr Package. *J. Stat. Softw.* **2021**, *99*, 1–36. [CrossRef]
49. Bridges, J.F.P.; Hauber, A.B.; Marshall, D.; Lloyd, A.; Prosser, L.A.; Regier, D.A.; Johnson, F.R.; Mauskopf, J. Conjoint Analysis Applications in Health—A Checklist: A Report of the ISPOR Good Research Practices for Conjoint Analysis Task Force. *Value Health* **2011**, *14*, 403–413. [CrossRef] [PubMed]
50. Ali, A.; Ali, S.; Khan, S.A.; Khan, D.M.; Abbas, K.; Khalil, A.; Manzoor, S.; Khalil, U. Sample Size Issues in Multilevel Logistic Regression Models. *PLoS ONE* **2019**, *14*, e0225427. [CrossRef] [PubMed]
51. McNeish, D. On Using Bayesian Methods to Address Small Sample Problems. *Struct. Equ. Model.* **2016**, *23*, 750–773. [CrossRef]
52. Smid, S.C.; McNeish, D.; Miočević, M.; van de Schoot, R. Bayesian Versus Frequentist Estimation for Structural Equation Models in Small Sample Contexts: A Systematic Review. *Struct. Equ. Model.* **2020**, *27*, 131–161. [CrossRef]
53. Regier, D.A.; Ryan, M.; Phimister, E.; Marra, C.A. Bayesian and Classical Estimation of Mixed Logit: An Application to Genetic Testing. *J. Health Econ.* **2009**, *28*, 598–610. [CrossRef] [PubMed]
54. Miočević, M.; Levy, R.; Schoot, R. van de Introduction to Bayesian Statistics. In *Small Sample Size Solutions*; Routledge: London, UK, 2020; ISBN 978-0-429-27387-2.
55. Depaoli, S.; van de Schoot, R. Improving Transparency and Replication in Bayesian Statistics: The WAMBS-Checklist. *Psychol. Methods* **2017**, *22*, 240–261. [CrossRef]
56. Aspinall, W. Structured Elicitation of Expert Judgment for Probabilistic Hazard and Risk Assessment in Volcanic Eruptions. In *Statistics in Volcanology*; Special Publications of IAVCEI, No. 1; Mader, H., Coles, S., Connor, C., Connor, L., Eds.; Geological Society of London: London, UK, 2006; pp. 15–30, ISBN 978-1-86239-208-3.
57. Würdemann, F.S.; Wilschut, J.A.; Hegeman, J.H. *Eindverslag SKMS Project Doorontwikkeling DHFA*; Dutch Institute for Clinical Auditing: Leiden, The Netherlands, 2021.
58. van Buuren, S.; Groothuis-Oudshoorn, K. Mice: Multivariate Imputation by Chained Equations in R. *J. Stat. Softw.* **2011**, *45*, 1–67. [CrossRef]
59. Hanea, A.M.; Nane, G.F. An In-Depth Perspective on the Classical Model. In *Expert Judgement in Risk and Decision Analysis*; Hanea, A.M., Nane, G.F., Bedford, T., French, S., Eds.; International Series in Operations Research & Management Science; Springer International Publishing: Cham, Switzerland, 2021; pp. 225–256, ISBN 978-3-030-46474-5.
60. Gilks, W.R. Markov Chain Monte Carlo. In *Encyclopedia of Biostatistics*; Armitage, P., Colton, T., Eds.; John Wiley & Sons, Ltd.: Hoboken, NJ, USA, 2005; ISBN 978-0-470-01181-2.
61. Martin, A.D.; Quinn, K.M.; Park, J.H. MCMCpack: Markov Chain Monte Carlo in R. *J. Stat. Softw.* **2011**, *42*, 1–21. [CrossRef]

62. Geweke, J.; In, F. Evaluating the Accuracy of Sampling-Based Approaches to the Calculation of Posterior Moments. 1995. Available online: https://www.researchgate.net/publication/2352607_Evaluating_the_Accuracy_of_Sampling-Based_Approaches_to_the_Calculation_of_Posterior_Moments (accessed on 8 March 2024).
63. de Bekker-Grob, E.W.; Donkers, B.; Jonker, M.F.; Stolk, E.A. Sample Size Requirements for Discrete-Choice Experiments in Healthcare: A Practical Guide. *Patient* **2015**, *8*, 373–384. [CrossRef] [PubMed]
64. Harrison, R.L. Introduction to Monte Carlo Simulation. *AIP Conf. Proc.* **2010**, *1204*, 17–21. [CrossRef] [PubMed]
65. Marti, D.; Mazzuchi, T.A.; Cooke, R.M. Are Performance Weights Beneficial? Investigating the Random Expert Hypothesis. In *Expert Judgement in Risk and Decision Analysis*; Hanea, A.M., Nane, G.F., Bedford, T., French, S., Eds.; International Series in Operations Research & Management Science; Springer International Publishing: Cham, Switzerland, 2021; pp. 53–82, ISBN 978-3-030-46474-5.
66. Spronk, I.; Loggers, S.A.I.; Joosse, P.; Willems, H.C.; Van Balen, R.; Gosens, T.; Ponsen, K.J.; Steens, J.; Van de Ree, L.C.P.; Zuurmond, R.G.; et al. Shared Decision-Making for the Treatment of Proximal Femoral Fractures in Frail Institutionalised Older Patients: Healthcare Providers' Perceived Barriers and Facilitators. *Age Ageing* **2022**, *51*, afac174. [CrossRef] [PubMed]
67. Sachs, G.A.; Shega, J.W.; Cox-Hayley, D. Barriers to Excellent End-of-Life Care for Patients with Dementia. *J. Gen. Intern. Med.* **2004**, *19*, 1057–1063. [CrossRef] [PubMed]
68. Mitchell, S.L.; Kiely, D.K.; Hamel, M.B. Dying with Advanced Dementia in the Nursing Home. *Arch. Intern. Med.* **2004**, *164*, 321–326. [CrossRef]
69. Ahronheim, J.C.; Morrison, R.S.; Baskin, S.A.; Morris, J.; Meier, D.E. Treatment of the Dying in the Acute Care Hospital. Advanced Dementia and Metastatic Cancer. *Arch. Intern. Med.* **1996**, *156*, 2094–2100. [CrossRef]
70. Boyd, K.; Murray, S.A. Recognising and Managing Key Transitions in End of Life Care. *BMJ* **2010**, *341*, c4863. [CrossRef]
71. Rurup, M.L.; Onwuteaka-Philipsen, B.D.; Pasman, H.R.W.; Ribbe, M.W.; van der Wal, G. Attitudes of Physicians, Nurses and Relatives towards End-of-Life Decisions Concerning Nursing Home Patients with Dementia. *Patient Educ. Couns.* **2006**, *61*, 372–380. [CrossRef]
72. Volicer, L.; Rheaume, Y.; Brown, J.; Fabiszewski, K.; Brady, R. Hospice Approach to the Treatment of Patients with Advanced Dementia of the Alzheimer Type. *JAMA* **1986**, *256*, 2210–2213. [CrossRef]
73. Sullivan, N.M.; Blake, L.E.; George, M.; Mears, S.C. Palliative Care in the Hip Fracture Patient. *Geriatr. Orthop. Surg. Rehabil.* **2019**, *10*, 2151459319849801. [CrossRef]
74. Yellen, S.B.; Cella, D.F.; Leslie, W.T. Age and Clinical Decision Making in Oncology Patients. *J. Natl. Cancer Inst.* **1994**, *86*, 1766–1770. [CrossRef] [PubMed]
75. Adamowicz, K.; Baczkowska-Waliszewska, Z. Quality of Life during Chemotherapy, Hormonotherapy or antiHER2 Therapy of Patients with Advanced, Metastatic Breast Cancer in Clinical Practice. *Health Qual. Life Outcomes* **2020**, *18*, 134. [CrossRef] [PubMed]
76. Falci, C.; Morello, E.; Droz, J.P. Treatment of Prostate Cancer in Unfit Senior Adult Patients. *Cancer Treat. Rev.* **2009**, *35*, 522–527. [CrossRef] [PubMed]
77. Hind, D.; Wyld, L.; Reed, M.W. Surgery, with or without Tamoxifen, vs Tamoxifen Alone for Older Women with Operable Breast Cancer: Cochrane Review. *Br. J. Cancer* **2007**, *96*, 1025–1029. [CrossRef]
78. Nijmeijer, W.S.; Voorthuis, B.J.; Groothuis-Oudshoorn, C.G.M.; Würdemann, F.S.; van der Velde, D.; Vollenbroek-Hutten, M.M.R.; Hegeman, J.H.; on behalf of the Dutch Hip Fracture Audit Taskforce Indicators Group. The Prediction of Early Mortality Following Hip Fracture Surgery in Patients Aged 90 Years and Older: The Almelo Hip Fracture Score 90 (AHFS90). *Osteoporos. Int.* **2023**, *34*, 867–877. [CrossRef]

Journal of
Clinical Medicine

MDPI

Article

The Impact of Implementation of Palliative, Non-Operative Management on Mortality of Operatively Treated Geriatric Hip Fracture Patients: A Retrospective Cohort Study

Thomas Nijdam *, Tim Schiepers, Duco Laane, Henk Jan Schuijt, Detlef van der Velde and Diederik Smeeing

Department of Trauma Surgery, St. Antonius Hospital Utrecht, 3543 AZ Utrecht, The Netherlands
* Correspondence: t.nijdam@antoniusziekenhuis.nl; Tel.: +31-63-833-4066

Abstract: (1) **Background:** Hip fracture patients with very limited life expectancy can opt for non-operative management (NOM) within a palliative care context. The implementation of NOM in the palliative context may affect the mortality of the operatively treated population. This retrospective cohort study aimed to determine whether the operatively treated geriatric hip fracture population would have a lower in-hospital mortality rate and fewer postoperative complications after the introduction of NOM within a palliative care context for patients with very limited life expectancy. (2) **Methods:** Data from 1 February 2019 to 1 February 2022 of patients aged 70 years or older were analyzed to give a comparison between patients before and after implementation of NOM within a palliative care context. (3) **Results:** Comparison between 550 patients before and 485 patients after implementation showed no significant difference in in-hospital or 1-year mortality rates (2.9% vs. 1.4%, $p = 0.139$; 22.4% vs. 20.2%, $p = 0.404$, respectively). Notably, post-implementation, fewer patients had prior dementia diagnoses (15% vs. 21%, $p = 0.010$), and intensive care unit admissions decreased (3.5% vs. 1.2%, $p = 0.025$). (4) **Conclusions:** The implementation of NOM within a palliative care context did not significantly reduce mortality or complications. However, NOM within palliative care is deemed a more patient-centered approach for geriatric hip fracture patients with very limited life expectancy.

Keywords: hip fracture; geriatric; mortality; complications; palliative; non-operative; operative

1. Introduction

Hip fractures in older patients are increasingly prevalent in current trauma care and create a rising problem, with the global number of hip fractures expected to increase to 6.3 million annually in 2050 [1,2]. Hip fractures are historically treated with operative management (OM); however, outcomes (i.e., mortality and morbidity) following OM remain very poor for specific phenotypes of geriatric patients with several risk factors associated with adverse outcomes [3–6]. These risk factors include increasing age, the American Society of Anesthesiologists (ASA) classification of three or higher, low ambulation status, and cognitive impairment [4,6]. For these frail geriatric hip fracture patients with very limited life expectancy, a new non-operative management (NOM) within a palliative care context is increasingly offered as an alternative to OM [7,8]. This differs from historical non-operative management, which was typically received by relatively young and healthy individuals with non-displaced femoral neck fractures, or those with significant comorbidities that rendered surgery non-beneficial, often leading to surgical refusal by the anesthesia team [7,9]. Therefore, NOM within a palliative care context encompasses a distinct form of non-operative treatment, different from the historical non-operative approach. With NOM within a palliative care context, patients can opt through shared decision-making (SDM) for a more peaceful last phase of life compared to an uncertain period of invasive rehabilitation after hip fracture surgery [10,11]. Current literature has focused on the mortality of the geriatric hip fracture population, including operatively treated patients with very limited life expectancy [12–15]. However, these mortality rates for geriatric hip fracture patients after OM could be skewed due to this group of frail patients with limited life expectancy. The hypothesis is that these patients, who only recently have other options than OM, influenced the previously reported mortality rate of the operatively treated hip fracture population and consequently made it appear worse. Therefore, after the introduction of NOM within a palliative care context, the operatively treated hip fracture population might show fewer adverse outcomes after OM, resulting in a decrease in the burden of care at the trauma-geriatric ward. This study aims to determine whether the operatively treated geriatric hip fracture population will have a lower in-hospital mortality rate and fewer postoperative complications after the introduction of NOM within a palliative care context.

2. Materials and Methods

2.1. Study Design

This retrospective cohort study was performed on geriatric hip fracture patients who presented to the emergency department (ED) of a large regional teaching hospital in the Netherlands between 1 February 2019 and 1 February 2022. Patients were identified from the electronic medical records through Diagnosis Related Groups (abbreviated as Diagnose Behandel Combinatie in Dutch): 218, hip fracture. The Business Intelligence department utilized code 218 to extract patient identification codes for all hip fracture patients. Patients were eligible for inclusion if they were aged 70 years or older and were admitted to the trauma-geriatric ward after OM for a hip fracture. Patients with a pathological hip fracture, an injury severity score of 16 or higher, or a periprosthetic hip fracture were excluded. File searching was conducted on all eligible patients to gather variables essential for this study. The STROBE guidelines were used to guide this study [16].

2.2. Non-Operative Management within a Palliative Care Context

NOM within a palliative care context has emerged as a novel treatment approach with a distinct palliative perspective. Loggers et al. have demonstrated that patients opting for NOM within a palliative care context experience a quality of life that is non-inferior to that of individuals opting for surgical intervention during the terminal phases of life; indicating NOM as a viable treatment strategy within palliative care settings, emphasizing a more patient-centered approach [11].

NOM within a palliative care context was introduced in this center as an option on 1 August 2020 for geriatric hip fracture patients considered frail and with very limited life expectancy. Patients were considered frail with one or more frailty criteria (body mass index (BMI) of 18.5 kg/m^2 or lower, functional ambulation category (FAC) of 2 or lower pre-trauma, ASA score of 4 or 5) or on the clinical judgment of the attending surgeon when thought of limited life expectancy without meeting the frailty criteria [11]. This clinical judgment is informed by the intuition of highly experienced trauma surgeons who frequently encounter such patients. The option is presented through an extensive shared decision-making (SDM) conversation, frequently involving family members, wherein both the outcomes of surgery and NOM within a palliative care context are thoroughly discussed. Approximately 25% of patients presenting to the ED engage in an extensive shared decision-making conversation, during which both treatment options are thoroughly discussed. Ultimately, approximately half of these patients choose NOM within a palliative care context, while the remaining half express a preference for surgical intervention. Hence, patients always retain the option to undergo surgery if they wish to. With NOM within a palliative care context, specific attention is paid to analgesia and patient comfort without aiming the patient to regain mobility and start the active rehabilitation program [11]. With the emergence of new effective analgesic modalities, such as the pericapsular nerve group block, a peripheral nerve block, satisfactory results regarding patient comfort ought to be achieved [17]. Since NOM within a palliative care context is not curative management, patients are likely to die within weeks after hip fracture (median survival 11 days

(IQR 4-26)) [10]. The renewed hip fracture pathway for geriatric patients is shown in Supplemental Figure S1.

2.3. Study Variables

The following baseline characteristics were collected from electronic medical records: age, sex, prior diagnosis of dementia (diagnosed by a geriatrician or general practitioner), BMI, Charlson Comorbidity Index (CCI), pre-fracture living situation (independent at home, at home with assistance for activities of daily living, institutionalized care facility), pre-fracture mobility (freely mobile without aids, mobile with one aid, mobile with two aids or frame, indoor mobility but outdoor immobile, no functional mobility), type of fracture (based on the OTA classification: OTA 31A for trochanteric fractures or OTA 31B for femoral neck fractures), and type of surgical procedure (sliding hip screw, proximal femoral nail anti-rotation, hemiarthroplasty, cannulated hip screw, hip arthroplasty) [18].

2.4. Outcome Measures

The primary outcome of this study was in-hospital mortality. Secondary outcomes were postoperative complications (surgical and non-surgical complications), admission to an intensive care unit (ICU), hospital length of stay, hospital readmission within 30 days after discharge, 30-day mortality, 90-day mortality, and 1-year mortality. Surgical complications included wound infection, postoperative hemorrhage, or secondary surgical intervention, such as wound rinsing and prosthesis revision. Non-operative complications included thrombo-embolic events (cerebrovascular accidents, deep venous thrombosis, and pulmonary embolisms), cardiac complications (myocardial infarction, arrhythmia, and congestive heart failure), pneumonia, urinary tract infection, delirium, pressure ulcer, need for blood transfusion, and urinary retention. Data on mortality were acquired by consulting the municipal citizen registry, and data on complications, when diagnosed by an attending physician, were extracted from electronic medical records.

2.5. Statistical Analysis

Statistical analysis was performed using SPSS for Windows 20.0 (IBM, Chicago, IL, USA). Differences between patients admitted before (pre-cohort) and after (post-cohort) the implementation of NOM within a palliative care context were analyzed using descriptive statistics. Continuous variables were tested for differences between groups with an unpaired t-test or Mann–Whitney U test, depending on normality. Normality was tested using the Shapiro–Wilk test. All categorical and dichotomous data were tested with a chi-square test. Descriptive statistics have been presented as mean with standard deviation or median with interquartile ranges (IQRs), depending on the distribution. For all statistical tests, p-values less than or equal to 0.05 are considered significant.

3. Results

3.1. Patient Demographics

In total, 1263 patients presented at the ED with a hip fracture. After exclusion, 1035 were included in the analysis. A total of 550 patients were included in the pre-cohort, and 485 patients were included in the post-cohort (Figure 1). The study population had a median age of 82 years (IQR 76–87), consisted of 688 females (66.5%), and had a median BMI of 24.0 (IQR 21.7–26.7). A femoral neck fracture was diagnosed in 588 (56.8%) of the patients, whereas 447 (43.2%) patients sustained a trochanteric fracture. The majority of 666 patients (64.3%) lived independently at home without additional care before admission, 206 patients (19.9%) lived at home with activities for daily living (ADL) support, and 163 patients (15.7%) were admitted to an institutionalized care facility (Table 1). Regarding the patients who were excluded from this analysis for receiving NOM within a palliative care context, these patients (n = 71) had a median age of 86 (IQR 82–91), 46 (64.8%) were female, 43 (60.6%) had a prior diagnosis of dementia, and the median CCI was 6 (IQR 5–7).

Prior to the fracture, 46 (64.8%) patients lived in an institutionalized care facility, and only 4 (5.6%) patients could mobilize freely without aids (Table 2).

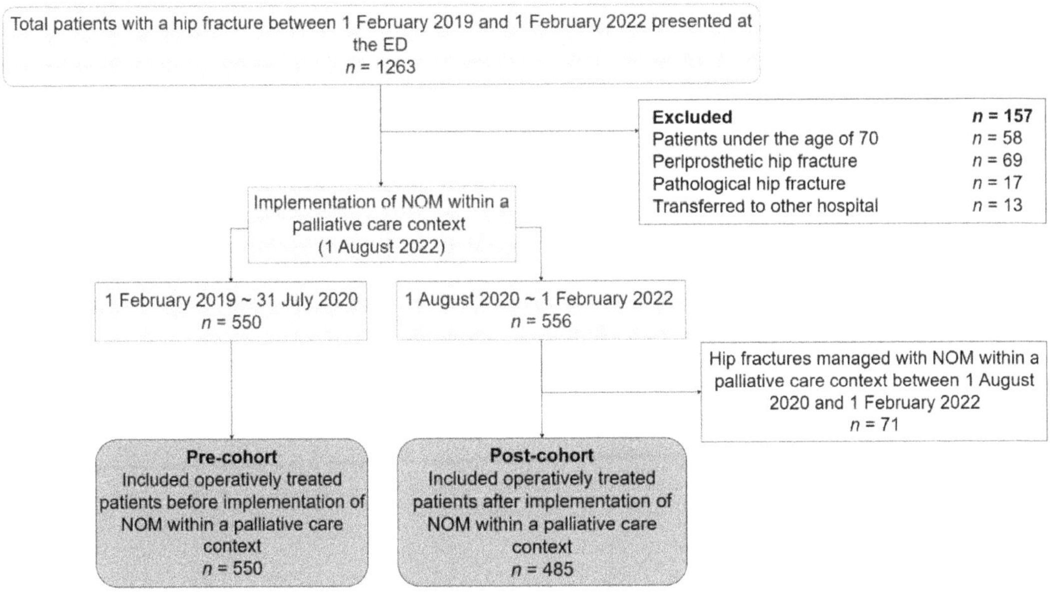

Figure 1. Flow chart of the selection process of included patients who underwent operative treatment for a hip fracture. ED = emergency department; NOM = non-operative management.

Table 1. Baseline characteristics of hip fracture patients who underwent operative treatment.

Baseline Variable	Data Missing	Total (n = 1035)	Pre-Cohort (n = 550)	Post-Cohort (n = 485)	p-Value
Age (in years)	0 (0)	82 (76–87)	82 (77–88)	82 (76–87)	0.893
Female sex	0 (0)	688 (66.5)	379 (68.9)	309 (63.7)	0.086
Prior diagnosis of dementia	0 (0)	188 (18.2)	116 (21.1)	72 (14.8)	0.010
BMI in kg/m^2	27 (2.6)	24.0 (21.7–26.7)	23.9 (21.6–26.2)	24.2 (21.9–27.0)	0.095
CCI	0 (0)	5 (4–6)	5 (4–6)	5 (4–6)	0.373
Living situation before fracture	0 (0)				0.151
Home, independent		666 (64.3)	341 (62.0)	325 (67.0)	
Home, with ADL care		206 (20.0)	112 (20.4)	94 (19.4)	
Institutionalized care facility		163 (15.7)	97 (17.6)	66 (13.6)	
Pre-fracture mobility	2 (0.2)				0.147
Freely without aids		467 (45.1)	243 (44.2)	224 (46.2)	
Outdoors with 1 aid		47 (4.6)	27 (4.9)	20 (4.1)	
Outdoors with 2 aids or frame		496 (47.9)	272 (49.5)	224 (46.2)	
Indoor, but immobile outside		18 (1.7)	4 (0.7)	14 (2.9)	
No functional mobility		5 (0.5)	3 (0.5)	2 (0.4)	
Fracture type	0 (0)				0.314
Femoral neck fracture		588 (56.8)	304 (55.3)	284 (58.6)	
Trochanteric fracture		447 (43.2)	246 (44.7)	201 (41.4)	

Table 1. *Cont.*

Baseline Variable	Data Missing	Total (*n* = 1035)	Pre-Cohort (*n* = 550)	Post-Cohort (*n* = 485)	*p*-Value
Surgical procedure	0 (0)				0.136
Sliding hip screw		69 (6.7)	41 (7.5)	28 (5.8)	
Proximal femoral nail anti-rotation		443 (42.8)	246 (44.7)	197 (40.6)	
Hemiarthroplasty		462 (44.6)	237 (43.1)	225 (46.4)	
Cannulated hip screw		6 (0.6)	4 (0.7)	2 (0.4)	
Total hip arthroplasty		55 (5.3)	22 (4.0)	33 (6.8)	

All variables are in total amount (percentage) or median (interquartile range, IQR). BMI = body mass index; CCI = Charlson Comorbidity Index; ADL = activities of daily living.

Table 2. Characteristics and outcomes of hip fracture patients who underwent non-operative management within a palliative care context.

NOM Cohort	Data Missing	Total (*n* = 71)
Age (in years)		86 (82–91)
Female sex		46 (64.8)
Prior diagnosis of dementia		43 (60.6)
BMI in kg/m^2	13 (18)	21.9 (19.7–24.2)
CCI		6 (5–7)
Living situation before fracture		
Home, independent		9 (12.7)
Home, with ADL care		16 (22.5)
Institutionalized care facility		46 (64.8)
Pre-fracture mobility	5 (7)	
Freely without aids		4 (5.6)
Outdoors with 1 aid		6 (8.5)
Outdoors with 2 aids or frame		29 (40.8)
Indoor, but immobile outside		19 (26.8)
No functional mobility		8 (11.2)
Admission in hospital		43 (60.6)
Hospital length of stay (in days)		3 (2–5)
Mortality		
In-hospital		8 (11.3)
30-day		57 (80.3)
90-day		63 (88.7)
1-year		68 (95.8)
Time till death (in days)		9 (5–22)

All variables are in total amount (percentage) or median (interquartile range, IQR). BMI = body mass index; CCI = Charlson Comorbidity Index; ADL = activities of daily living.

In the pre-cohort, 379 patients (68.9%) were female, and the post-cohort consisted of 309 female patients (63.7%) ($p = 0.086$). The post-cohort had significantly fewer patients diagnosed with dementia than the pre-cohort (72 (15%) vs. 116 (21%), $p = 0.010$). No significant difference between the pre-cohort and post-cohort was measured in the living situation and pre-fracture mobility before the hip fracture. In addition, there were no significant differences between the two cohorts at baseline regarding age, BMI, fracture type, or surgical procedure.

3.2. Mortality and Postoperative Complications

After the implementation of NOM within a palliative care context, no statistically significant difference was observed in in-hospital mortality (2.9% vs. 1.4%, p = 0.139). Additionally, the 30-day (6.4% vs. 4.7%, p = 0.281), 90-day (10.9% vs. 10.3%, p = 0.763), and 1-year (22.4% vs. 20.2%, p = 0.404) mortality follow-up periods also showed no statistical significance in mortality between the two cohorts (Table 3). Significantly more postoperative hemorrhages occurred in the post-cohort (0.2% vs. 1.9%, p = 0.018). Admissions to the ICU showed a significant decrease in the post-cohort (3.5% vs. 1.2%, p = 0.025). There were no significant differences in the incidence of other complications, readmissions, or hospital length of stay (Table 3). In total, 8 out of 71 (11.3%) patients died in the hospital who opted for NOM within a palliative care context. The 30-day, 90-day, and 1-year mortality were 57 (80.3%), 63 (88.7%), and 68 (95.8%), respectively. The median number of days until death for patients who opted for NOM within a palliative care context was 9 (IQR 5-22) days after hip fracture (Table 2).

Table 3. Patient outcomes of operatively treated hip fracture patients.

Patient Outcomes	Pre-Cohort (n = 550)	Post-Cohort (n = 485)	p-Value
Mortality			
In-hospital	16 (2.9)	7 (1.4)	0.139
30-day	35 (6.4)	23 (4.7)	0.281
90-day	60 (10.9)	50 (10.3)	0.763
1-year	123 (22.4)	98 (20.2)	0.402
Patients with complications	286 (52)	272 (56)	0.190
Surgical complications	28	31	
Wound infection	24 (4.4)	20 (4.1)	0.878
Secondary hemorrhage	1 (0.2)	9 (1.9)	0.018
Re-intervention	3 (0.5)	2 (0.4)	1.000
Non-surgical complications	418	416	
Thrombo-embolic	8 (1.5)	8 (1.6)	0.807
Cardiac	42 (7.6)	40 (8.2)	0.731
Pneumonia	48 (8.7)	41 (8.5)	0.912
UTI	37 (6.7)	35 (7.2)	0.807
Delirium	149 (27.1)	138 (28.5)	0.627
Pressure ulcer	26 (4.7)	30 (6.2)	0.336
Anemia	70 (12.7)	77 (15.9)	0.154
Urinary retention	30 (5.5)	40 (8.2)	0.083
Sepsis	8 (1.5)	7 (1.4)	1.000
Admission to ICU	19 (3.5)	8 (1.2)	0.025
Readmission	26 (4.7)	32 (6.6)	0.223
Hospital length of stay (in days)	6 (4-9)	6 (5-9)	0.053

All variables are in total amount (percentage) or median (interquartile range, IQR). UTI = urinary tract infection; ICU = intensive care unit.

4. Discussion

This study retrospectively analyzed elderly patients admitted to the trauma-geriatric ward after OM. The results of this study showed no significantly lower mortality rate or fewer postoperative complications for the post-cohort after the introduction of NOM within a palliative care context for hip fracture patients. However, significantly fewer operatively treated demented patients and significantly fewer ICU admissions in the post-cohort were observed. In addition, the NOM group showed the majority of patients opting for this management after hip fracture dying within 30 days (80.3%) with a median time till death of 9 (5–22) days.

This study observed an in-hospital mortality risk of 2.9% pre-implementation and 1.4% post-implementation, which corresponds with recent studies showing in-hospital mortality rates for geriatric hip fracture patients ranging from 1.5% to 5.0% [12,14,15]. Although the difference between the two cohorts in this study was not significant, a cautious trend to a lower in-hospital mortality can be seen in the percentage of in-hospital deceased patients. Subsequently, there are indications of a lower mortality rate with the absence of high-risk patients opting for NOM within a palliative care context. One-year mortality rates of 22.4% pre-implementation and 20.2% post-implementation also showed no significant decrease but did show lower mortality rates than recent literature, which ranges from 23.2% to 35.1% [19–22]. Compared with a 2018 cohort study in our center with a reported mortality rate of 27.0%, this study found substantially lower 1-year mortality rates [19]. This could be explained by the recent introduction of trauma-geriatric units and their subsequent improvement over the years [22–24]. One possible explanation for the minor impact on mortality rates could be that the clinical outcomes of the post-cohort were affected by the COVID-19 pandemic since these two periods largely coincided. The interference of the pandemic cannot be ruled out and possibly led to an overestimation of mortality, especially in the post-cohort since the geriatric population is particularly at risk of dying from COVID-19 [25–27]. Recent studies report that COVID-19 more than doubles the 90-day mortality rate following hip fracture and show a 30-day mortality rate of 34% in hip fracture patients with a COVID-19 infection [28,29]. Due to limitations in ascertaining the cause of death for patients who did not die within the hospital setting and privacy constraints that prevent access to such information from the municipal citizen registry, it was deemed unreliable to include these values in this study.

In the post-cohort (14.8%), there were significantly fewer patients with a prior diagnosis of dementia compared to the pre-cohort (21.1%). The incidence of the post-cohort is lower than earlier studies, showing an incidence of 20-28%, which is more in line with the incidence of the pre-cohort [19,24,30,31]. In recent literature, a high percentage (73%) of patients diagnosed with dementia opted for this NOM within a palliative care context after hip fracture, which probably explains the significant decrease in demented patients undergoing OM [10]. In a survey to investigate the general public's view on life-sustaining treatment in the case of dementia, 72.9% expressed a preference for a peaceful passing and 68.9% expressed a preference for their partner to have a peaceful passing [32]. Therefore, it is possible that patients with dementia or those who care for them are more likely to opt for NOM within a palliative care context.

Although dementia has also been identified as a risk factor for early mortality after hip fracture, this does not imply that all dementia patients are at high risk of adverse outcomes after OM since this is a heterogeneous population with a wide range of physical and cognitive conditions resulting in a variable outcome [33]. Therefore, in the dementia population, it remains essential to include individual risk assessments in the decision-making process.

A possible explanation that the post-cohort did not show fewer postoperative complications could be due to the introduction of an automated complication registration method in our hospital in January 2021, as it is previously studied that automation of the registration process results in a rise in the incidence of registered complications without the increase in relative complications [34].

The postoperative incidence of secondary hemorrhage even increased significantly in the post-cohort. This result may be due to an increase in the usage of direct oral anticoagulants (DOACs) over the last few years [35]. Using a DOAC will not result in an unnecessary surgical delay in our center. There is evidence that wound complications, including secondary hemorrhage, have a higher incidence in geriatric hip fracture patients using DOACs [36].

Contrarily, ICU admissions showed a significant decrease in the post-cohort to 1.2%, which is also lower than that of previously reported incidence rates of 3–4%, which is again more in line with the incidence of the pre-cohort of 3.5% [30,37]. It seems possible that the incidence of patients with severe adverse outcomes requiring ICU admission after OM significantly decreased due to the identification of frail patients performed in acute settings resulting in a decrease in OM in the frailest patients. However, as previously stated, the post-cohort largely coincided with the COVID-19 pandemic. Therefore, it is important to consider that the decrease in ICU admissions during this period may be attributable to the limited availability of ICU beds; consequently, reducing the proportion of geriatric hip fractures admitted to the ICU [38].

One of the strengths of this study, since NOM within a palliative care context is relatively new in hip fracture management, is being the first to investigate the impact of the introduction of NOM within a palliative care context on operatively treated hip fracture patients in terms of mortality and morbidity. The main limitation was this study's retrospective nature, resulting in difficulty in acquiring follow-up data for geriatric patient populations and, therefore, minor complications after admission or cause of death. Consequently, information on postoperative outcomes after discharge was only available if patients revisited the hospital. Furthermore, an additional limitation arises due to the inherent variability in treatment techniques for hip fractures, which depend on numerous fracture- and patient-related factors These variations may lead to differences in postoperative rehabilitation protocols and complication rates. Nevertheless, we opted to analyze the operatively treated group as a whole because our primary objective was to assess whether the overall cohort was influenced by the inclusion of very frail geriatric patients who likely opted for NOM within a palliative care context since its implementation. Another limitation could be the possible underpowering of this study due to the limited amount of available data post-implementation. However, this study has described the largest possible patient cohort following the implementation of NOM within a palliative care context in this center, representing the most comprehensive dataset within the specified timeframe. In addition, changes in management and protocols over time could also have affected the primary and secondary outcomes. Therefore, potential confounding due to the effect of time could exist. Lastly, this study only collected clinical data as outcome measures without functional or psychological outcomes. Future studies with prospective designs could give more insights into a possible improvement in these outcomes.

With the results of this study, it is tempting to speculate that in the post-cohort, there is no direct decrease in the overall frailty of the operatively treated hip fracture population. A decrease in total numbers was described; however not a statistically significant decrease in in-hospital mortality, there are indications that those with a high risk of short-term adverse outcomes are more likely to opt for NOM within a palliative care context. Furthermore, since patients opting for NOM within a palliative care context stay significantly shorter in the hospital and often (35.0%) return directly from the ED to their place of origin, fewer complex hip fracture patients are admitted to the trauma-geriatric ward, which further decreases the burden of care [11]. It is worth mentioning that although costs should not influence the choice of treatment, the introduction of NOM within a palliative care context has significantly lowered healthcare costs compared to OM, primarily due to shorter median hospital length of stay (3 (IQR 2–5) vs. 6 (IQR 4–9) days) and costs related to surgery and readmissions [39]. However, most importantly, with the introduction of NOM within a palliative care context, a shift in thinking from a disease-oriented to a patient-goal-oriented paradigm is ensured. This will provide better person-centered care for geriatric patients with limited life expectancy.

5. Conclusions

The introduction of NOM within a palliative care context for geriatric hip fracture patients did not result in a significantly lower in-hospital mortality rate, fewer postoperative complications, and hospital readmissions in the surgically treated geriatric hip fracture population. However, NOM within a palliative care context is considered a more patient-centered treatment modality by frail geriatric hip fracture patients with reduced pre-fracture mobility and very limited life expectancy.

Supplementary Materials: The following supporting information can be downloaded at https://www.mdpi.com/article/10.3390/jcm13072012/s1, Figure S1: Renewed hip fracture pathway for geriatric patients.

Author Contributions: D.v.d.V. was the guarantor of this study and made substantial contributions to the concept together with H.J.S. and D.S., T.N. and T.S. contributed equally to the data collection and statistical analyses and had both major contributions in writing the manuscript along with D.L. All authors worked on the interpretation of the data, contributed to intellectual content, and approved the final version of the manuscript to be published. All authors have read and agreed to the published version of the manuscript.

Funding: This research received no external funding.

Institutional Review Board Statement: The study was conducted in accordance with the principles outlined in the Declaration of Helsinki and Good Clinical Practice (GCP), and the Medical Ethics Committee, Utrecht (MEC-U), The Netherlands (W22.101), approved the study design on 18 May 2022.

Informed Consent Statement: Due to the retrospective design of the study and its involved file research, the executive board of the MEC-U considered that there is no violation of physical or psychological integrity; therefore, the ethical committee deemed no informed consent necessary.

Data Availability Statement: The datasets used and/or analyzed during the current study are available from the corresponding author upon reasonable request.

Conflicts of Interest: The authors declare no conflicts of interest.

References

1. Cheng, S.Y.; Levy, A.R.; Lefaivre, K.A.; Guy, P.; Kuramoto, L.; Sobolev, B. Geographic trends in incidence of hip fractures A comprehensive literature review. *Osteoporos Int.* **2011**, *22*, 2575–2586. [CrossRef] [PubMed]
2. Cooper, C.; Campion, G.; Melton, L.J. Hip fractures in the elderly: A world-wide projection. *Osteoporos Int.* **1992**, *2*, 285–289 [CrossRef] [PubMed]
3. Nkanang, B.; Parker, M.; Parker, E.; Griffiths, R. Perioperative mortality for patients with a hip fracture. *Injury* **2017**, *48*, 2180–2183 [CrossRef] [PubMed]
4. Chen, D.X.; Yang, L.; Ding, L.; Li, S.Y.; Qi, Y.N.; Li, Q. Perioperative outcomes in geriatric patients undergoing hip fracture surgery with different anesthesia techniques: A systematic review and meta-analysis. *Medicine* **2019**, *98*, e18220. [CrossRef] [PubMed]
5. Dizdarevic, A.; Farah, F.; Ding, J.; Shah, S.; Bryan, A.; Kahn, M.; Kaye, A.D.; Gritsenko, K. A Comprehensive Review of Analgesia and Pain Modalities in Hip Fracture Pathogenesis. *Curr. Pain Headache Rep.* **2019**, *23*, 72. [CrossRef] [PubMed]
6. Bentler, S.E.; Liu, L.; Obrizan, M.; Cook, E.A.; Wright, K.B.; Geweke, J.F.; Chrischilles, E.A.; Pavlik, C.E.; Wallace, R.B.; Ohsfeldt R.L.; et al. The aftermath of hip fracture: Discharge placement, functional status change, and mortality. *Am. J. Epidemiol.* **2009**, *170*, 1290–1299. [CrossRef] [PubMed]
7. Cram, P.; Yan, L.; Bohm, E.; Kuzyk, P.; Lix, L.M.; Morin, S.N.; Majumdar, S.R.; Leslie, W.D. Trends in Operative and Nonoperative Hip Fracture Management 1990–2014: A Longitudinal Analysis of Manitoba Administrative Data. *J. Am. Geriatr. Soc.* **2017**, *65* 27–34. [CrossRef] [PubMed]
8. Ko, F.C.; Morrison, R.S. A trigger for palliative care in vulnerable older adults. *JAMA Intern. Med.* **2014**, *174*, 1281–1282. [CrossRef] [PubMed]
9. Neuman, M.D.; Fleisher, L.A.; Even-Shoshan, O.; Mi, L.; Silber, J.H. Nonoperative care for hip fracture in the elderly: The influence of race, income, and comorbidities. *Med. Care* **2010**, *48*, 314–320. [CrossRef]
10. Nijdam, T.M.P.; Laane, D.W.P.M.; Spierings, J.F.; Schuijt, H.J.; Smeeing, D.P.J.; van der Velde, D. Proxy-reported experiences of palliative, non-operative management of geriatric patients after a hip fracture: A qualitative study. *BMJ Open* **2022**, *12*, e063007 [CrossRef] [PubMed]
11. Loggers, S.A.I.; Willems, H.C.; Van Balen, R.; Gosens, T.; Polinder, S.; Ponsen, K.J.; Van de Ree, C.L.P.; Steens, J.; Verhofstad M.H.J.; Zuurmond, R.G.; et al. Evaluation of Quality of Life after Nonoperative or Operative Management of Proximal Femoral Fractures in Frail Institutionalized Patients: The FRAIL-HIP Study. *JAMA Surg.* **2022**, *157*, 424–434. [CrossRef] [PubMed]
12. Groff, H.; Kheir, M.M.; George, J.; Azboy, I.; Higuera, C.A.; Parvizi, J. Causes of in-hospital mortality after hip fractures in the elderly. *HIP Int.* **2020**, *30*, 204–209. [CrossRef] [PubMed]
13. Sanz-Reig, J.; Salvador Marín, J.; Pérez Alba, J.M.; Ferrández Martínez, J.; Orozco Beltrán, D.; Martínez López, J.F. Risk factors for in-hospital mortality following hip fracture. *Rev. Española Cirugía Ortopédica Traumatol. Engl. Ed.* **2017**, *61*, 209–215. [CrossRef]

14. Erickson, B.J.; Nwachukwu, B.U.; Kiriakopoulos, E.; Frank, R.M.; Levine, B.; Villarroel, L.; Mccormick, F.M. In-hospital mortality risk for femoral neck fractures among patients receiving medicare. *Orthopedics* **2015**, *38*, e593–e596. [CrossRef] [PubMed]
15. Friedman, S.M.; Mendelson, D.A.; Bingham, K.W.; Kates, S.L. Impact of a comanaged geriatric fracture center on short-term hip fracture outcomes. *Arch. Intern. Med.* **2009**, *169*, 1712–1717. [CrossRef] [PubMed]
16. Cuschieri, S. The STROBE guidelines. *Saudi J. Anaesth.* **2019**, *13* (Suppl. S1), 31–34. [CrossRef] [PubMed]
17. Girón-Arango, L.; Peng, P.W.H.; Chin, K.J.; Brull, R.; Perlas, A. Pericapsular Nerve Group (PENG) Block for Hip Fracture. *Reg. Anesth. Pain Med.* **2018**, *43*, 859–863. [CrossRef] [PubMed]
18. Femur, B. Femur. *J. Orthop. Trauma* **2018**, *32*, S33–S44. [CrossRef]
19. Schuijt, H.J.; Kusen, J.; van Hernen, J.J.; van der Vet, P.; Geraghty, O.; Smeeing, D.P.J.; van der Velde, D. Orthogeriatric Trauma Unit Improves Patient Outcomes in Geriatric Hip Fracture Patients. *Geriatr. Orthop. Surg. Rehabil.* **2020**, *11*. [CrossRef] [PubMed]
20. Tarazona-Santabalbina, F.J.; Belenguer-Varea, Á.; Rovira-Daudi, E.; Salcedo-Mahiques, E.; Cuesta-Peredó, D.; Doménech-Pascual, J.R.; Salvador-Pérez, M.I.; Avellana-Zaragoza, J.A. Early interdisciplinary hospital intervention for elderly patients with hip fractures—Functional outcome and mortality. *Clinics* **2012**, *67*, 547–555. [CrossRef] [PubMed]
21. Lee, T.C.; Ho, P.S.; Lin, H.T.; Ho, M.L.; Huang, H.T.; Chang, J.K. One-year readmission risk and mortality after hip fracture surgery: A national population-based study in Taiwan. *Aging Dis.* **2017**, *8*, 402–409. [CrossRef] [PubMed]
22. Folbert, E.C.; Hegeman, J.H.; Vermeer, M.; Regtuijt, E.M.; van der Velde, D.; ten Duis, H.J.; Slaets, J.P. Improved 1-year mortality in elderly patients with a hip fracture following integrated orthogeriatric treatment. *Osteoporos Int.* **2017**, *28*, 269–277. [CrossRef] [PubMed]
23. Patel, J.N.; Klein, D.S.; Sreekumar, S.; Liporace, F.A.; Yoon, R.S. Outcomes in Multidisciplinary Team-based Approach in Geriatric Hip Fracture Care: A Systematic Review. *J. Am. Acad. Orthop. Surg.* **2020**, *28*, 128–133. [CrossRef] [PubMed]
24. Vidán, M.; Serra, J.A.; Moreno, C.; Riquelme, G.; Ortiz, J. Efficacy of a comprehensive geriatric intervention in older patients hospitalized for hip fracture: A randomized, controlled trial. *J. Am. Geriatr. Soc.* **2005**, *53*, 1476–1482. [CrossRef] [PubMed]
25. Becerra-Muñoz, V.M.; Núñez-Gil, I.J.; Eid, C.M.; Garciá Aguado, M.; Romero, R.; Huang, J.; Mulet, A.; Ugo, F.; Rametta, F.; Liebetrau, C.; et al. Clinical profile and predictors of in-hospital mortality among older patients hospitalised for COVID-19. *Age Ageing* **2021**, *50*, 326–334. [CrossRef] [PubMed]
26. Smits, R.A.L.; Trompet, S.; Van Der Linden, C.M.J.; Van Der Bol, J.M.; Jansen, S.W.M.; Polinder-Bos, H.A.; Willems, H.C.; Barten, D.G.; Blomaard, L.C.; de Boer, M.G.J.; et al. Characteristics and outcomes of older patients hospitalised for COVID-19 in the first and second wave of the pandemic in the Netherlands: The COVID-OLD study. *Age Ageing* **2022**, *51*, afac048. [CrossRef] [PubMed]
27. Lithander, F.E.; Neumann, S.; Tenison, E.; Lloyd, K.; Welsh, T.J.; Rodrigues, J.C.L.; Higgins, J.P.T.; Scourfield, L.; Christensen, H.; Haunton, V.J.; et al. COVID-19 in older people: A rapid clinical review. *Age Ageing* **2020**, *49*, 501–515. [CrossRef] [PubMed]
28. Holleyman, R.J.; Khan, S.K.; Charlett, A.; Inman, D.S.; Johansen, A.; Brown, C.; Barnard, S.; Fox, S.; Baker, P.N.; Deehan, D.; et al. The impact of COVID-19 on mortality after hip fracture: A population cohort study from England. *Bone Jt. J.* **2022**, *104-B*, 1156–1167. [CrossRef] [PubMed]
29. Alcock, H.; Moppett, E.A.; Moppett, I.K. Early mortality outcomes of patients with fragility hip fracture and concurrent SARS-CoV-2 infection a systematic review and meta-analysis. *Bone Jt. Open* **2021**, *2*, 314–322. [CrossRef] [PubMed]
30. Panula, J.; Pihlajamäki, H.; Mattila, V.M.; Jaatinen, P.; Vahlberg, T.; Aarnio, P.; Kivelä, S.-L. Mortality and cause of death in hip fracture patients aged 65 or older—A population-based study. *BMC Musculoskelet. Disord.* **2011**, *12*, 105. [CrossRef]
31. Tanner, A.; Jarvis, S.; Orlando, A.; Nwafo, N.; Madayag, R.; Roberts, Z.; Corrigan, C.; Carrick, M.; Bourg, P.; Smith, W.; et al. A three-year retrospective multi-center study on time to surgery and mortality for isolated geriatric hip fractures. *J. Clin. Orthop. Trauma* **2020**, *11*, S56–S61. [CrossRef] [PubMed]
32. Williams, N.; Dunford, C.; Knowles, A.; Warner, J. Public attitudes to life-sustaining treatments and euthanasia in dementia. *Int. J. Geriatr. Psychiatry* **2007**, *22*, 1229–1234. [CrossRef]
33. Deardorff, W.J.; Barnes, D.E.; Jeon, S.Y.; Boscardin, W.J.; Langa, K.M.; Covinsky, K.E.; Mitchell, S.L.; Whitlock, E.L.; Smith, A.K.; Lee, S.J. Development and External Validation of a Mortality Prediction Model for Community-Dwelling Older Adults with Dementia. *JAMA Intern. Med.* **2022**, *182*, 1161–1170. [CrossRef] [PubMed]
34. Veen, E.J.; Janssen-Heijnen, M.L.G.; Leenen, L.P.H.; Roukema, J.A. The registration of complications in surgery: A learning curve. *World J. Surg.* **2005**, *29*, 402–409. [CrossRef] [PubMed]
35. de Jong, L.A.; Koops, M.; Gout-Zwart, J.J.; Beinema, M.J.; Hemels, M.E.W.; Postma, M.J.; Brouwers, J.R.B.J. Trends in direct oral anticoagulant (DOAC) use: Health benefits and patient preference. *Neth. J. Med.* **2018**, *76*, 426–430. [PubMed]
36. Matheron, G.; Looby, I.; Khan, M.; Fazal, M.A. Novel Anticoagulants and Hip Fractures in the Elderly. *Cureus* **2022**, *14*, e23020. [CrossRef] [PubMed]
37. Donegan, D.J.; Gay, A.N.; Baldwin, K.; Morales, E.E.; Esterhai, J.L.; Mehta, S. Use of medical comorbidities to predict complications after hip fracture surgery in the elderly. *J. Bone Jt. Surg.* **2010**, *92*, 807–813. [CrossRef] [PubMed]

38. Arabi, Y.M.; Myatra, S.N.; Lobo, S.M. Surging ICU during COVID-19 pandemic: An overview. *Curr. Opin. Crit. Care* **2022**, *28*, 638–644. [CrossRef]
39. Loggers, S.A.I.; Geraerds, A.J.L.M.; Joosse, P.; Willems, H.C.; Gosens, T.; Van Balen, R.; Van de Ree, C.P.; Ponsen, K.J.; Steens, J.; Zuurmond, R.G.; et al. Nonoperative versus operative management of frail institutionalized older patients with a proximal femoral fracture: A cost-utility analysis alongside a multicenter prospective cohort study. *Osteoporos Int.* **2023**, *34*, 515–525. [CrossRef] [PubMed]

Journal of
Clinical Medicine

MDPI

Article

Beyond Mortality: Severely Frail Femur Fracture Patients Can Regain Independence after Surgery

Noa H. M. Ponds [1,2], Jochem H. Raats [1,2], Devon T. Brameier [1], Henk Jan Schuijt [3], Lisa Cooper [4,5], Abigail Sagona [1], Houman Javedan [4] and Michael J. Weaver [1,*]

1 Department of Orthopedic Surgery, Brigham and Women's Hospital, Harvard Medical School, Boston, MA 02215, USA
2 Department of Surgery, St. Antonius Hospital, 3543 AZ Utrecht, The Netherlands
3 Center for Geriatric Trauma, St. Antonius Hospital, 3543 AZ Utrecht, The Netherlands
4 Division of Aging, Department of Medicine, Brigham and Women's Hospital, Harvard Medical School, Boston, MA 02215, USA
5 Department of Geriatric Medicine, Rabin Medical Center, Tel Aviv 4941492, Israel
* Correspondence: mjweaver@bwh.harvard.edu; Tel.: +1-617-525-8088

Abstract: Objectives: Little is known about the post-operative functional outcomes of severely frail femur fracture patients, with previous studies focusing on complications and mortality. This study investigated patient- or proxy-reported outcomes after femur fracture surgery in older adult patients with severe frailty. **Methods:** This was a retrospective cross-sectional study of older adult (>70 years) patients with severe frailty (defined by a Comprehensive Geriatric Assessment-based Frailty Index (FI-CGA) $\geq$ 0.40), who underwent femur fracture surgery at a Level 1 Trauma Center. Patients or their proxy (i.e., close relative) reported mobility, psychosocial, and functional outcomes at least 1-year after surgery. **Results:** Thirty-seven predominantly female (76%) patients with a median age of 85 years (IQR 79–92), and a median FI-CGA of 0.48 (IQR 0.43–0.54) were included. Eleven patients (30%) regained pre-fracture levels of ambulation, with twenty-six patients (70%) able to walk with or without assistance. The majority of patients (76%) were able to have meaningful conversations. Of the patients, 54% of them experienced no to minimal pain, while 8% still experienced a lot of pain. Functional independence varied, as follows: five patients (14%) could bathe themselves; nine patients (25%) could dress themselves; fourteen patients (39%) could toilet independently; and seventeen patients (47%) transferred out of a (wheel)chair independently. **Conclusions:** Despite the high risk of mortality and perioperative complications, many of the most severely frail patients with surgically treated femur fractures regain the ability to ambulate and live with a moderate degree of independence. This information can help healthcare providers to better inform these patients and their families of the role of surgical treatment during goals of care discussions.

Keywords: geriatric trauma; femur fracture; frailty; self-reported outcome

1. Introduction

Increasing life expectancy and advancements in healthcare has resulted in a rise in the number of older adult patients presenting with a hip or femur fracture, as well as an increase in the degree of frailty these patients are living with [1,2]. Frailty is a dynamic biopsychosocial syndrome characterized by a decreased reserve to regain homeostasis after a stressor event. This is due to a pooled decline of multiple domains (including among them genetics, biology, function, cognition, nutrition, psychosocial well-being, and socio-economic status), leading to an inability to recover to baseline and, thus, a greater vulnerability and decreased resilience to adverse events such as falls, fractures, institutionalization, and death [3–8]. Among patients who suffer hip fractures, frailty has been associated with a higher risk of perioperative complications and mortality [9–11]. As a result, these frail patients require greater attention from both orthopedic surgeons and geriatricians, demanding multiple medical consultations to manage their many comorbidities. These patients often have extended lengths of stay (LOS), delayed surgery, and ultimately increased mortality [12–15]. Patients with severe frailty are entering a slow decline and approaching the end of their life. When managing femur fractures in these patients, it becomes increasingly important to balance expectations and benefits of surgery with the possible harm of surgical treatment, aligning patients' goals of care with expected outcomes.

Multidisciplinary management and treatment approaches, such as Orthogeriatric Co-management (OGC), have been shown to improve the outcomes and reduce the economic healthcare burden of geriatric fractures [11,16]. Frailty indices have been developed in an attempt to better capture patients' overall medical condition by accounting for age, medical comorbidities, and their functional and cognitive status. One example is the Comprehensive Geriatric Assessment (CGA)-based Frailty Index (FI-CGA), which assesses frailty in older adults by accounting for the accumulation of deficits and reserves based on variables collected during the CGA [17,18]. This includes (but is not limited to) patient-reported variables such as mood, changes in memory, polypharmacy, comorbidities, and functional variables [19]. The FI-CGA better predicts outcomes based on patients' physiological age as opposed to chronological age, with higher FI-CGA scores reflecting a higher risk for adverse outcomes and mortality [20–24].

There is a paucity of literature surrounding the long-term patient-reported outcomes of severely frail patients undergoing femur fracture surgery. Prior studies have focused on post-operative complications and mortality in these patients [25–27]. As this population often faces cognitive impairment, end-of-life care, and a continuous functional decline regardless of their injury, collecting appropriate functional measures is challenging. This difficulty has limited the available literature on this population, leading to these patients being assumed to face inevitable short-term mortality and poor patient outcomes following femur fractures [28]. In order to improve shared decision-making, it is important to understand the expected patient-centered outcomes of this specific population to inform goals of care discussions, and to align the expectations of patients and their families.

The objective of this study is to evaluate the functional outcomes of severely frail patients with femur fractures in terms of ambulatory status, pain relief, and activities of daily living.

2. Materials and Methods

This is a single-center, retrospective, cross-sectional study assessing the long-term functional outcomes of all consecutive severely frail older adult patients with surgically treated femur fractures (AO 31–33 A-C, including periprosthetic femur fractures) [29,30] over a 3-year period.

Patients were identified from electronic patient databases using the International Classification of Diseases Clinical Modification (ICD-CM) fracture codes (S72.0–S72.9) [31] and a review of their Electronic Health Record (EHR). Inclusion criteria were severely frail geriatric patients (as determined by having a FI-CGA ≥ 0.4 and an age of 70 years or older) with a surgically managed femur fracture, at least 1-year of follow-up, and a completed CGA by a geriatrician prior to their surgery with a calculated FI-CGA.

Eligible patients or proxies of patients were called and surveyed about patient-reported outcomes at what they considered the best point in the patient's recovery after surgery, in terms of functional ability. This patient-specific "best point in their recovery" was utilized as the time-point for measuring peak functional outcomes because the goal was to capture the maximal functional benefit gained from surgery in a population of patients who are in a constant physiological decline. As the rate of decline may vary from patient-to-patient, a patient-specific time-point for the "best point in their recovery" was selected as more appropriate for the outcomes of interest than an arbitrary single time-point in the recovery period. If patients were discharged to an institution and the patient or proxy could not be reached directly, the institution was called to make an attempt of contact with the patient or proxy. Patients were excluded if there was no response from the patient and/or proxy after a maximum of 3 attempts of contact, or if follow-up data (i.e., deceased and/or no available proxy, or no available information from the discharge institution) were not available.

In the study institution, a CGA is performed by geriatricians as part of the standard of care for all femur fracture patients aged 70 and above. The CGA is a multi-domain assessment of aging which includes cognitive, functional, and social assessments, in addition to a medication review and physical examination [19]. Information on all healthcare domains included in the calculation of the frailty index are collected within the CGA, which is then used to calculate an index score (FI-CGA) based on a deficit accumulation model of frailty, by using an integrated algorithm within the EHR as described elsewhere [17,18]. Frailty is defined as having a FI-CGA of 0.2 or higher. It has been shown that a FI-CGA $\geq$ 0.41 is associated with more cognitive and functional impairment. Greater frailty also showed a clear dose-dependent relationship (more = worse) with respect to community and ambulatory service use [18]. Moreover, a FI-CGA > 0.45 is related to higher mortality in community-dwelling adults [24].

In this study, a FI-CGA $\geq$ 0.4 was used to define severe frailty. A typical patient with an FI of 0.4 would be cognitively impaired, dependent on aids and/or others in terms of mobility and ADLs, and have a limited life expectancy. Most patients either live in an assisted living environment, or are close to needing that level of care. That being said, the severely frail patient population is very heterogenous in characteristics and outcomes, as dependency can manifest in all different domains of life.

Patient- or proxy-reported outcomes were chosen to reflect the absolute minimum requirements for a life with acceptable quality. Subjects were asked to recall the best point of the patients' recovery in terms of mobility, psychosocial, and functional outcomes. Mobility outcomes were assessed by ambulatory status (i.e., independent, with a walking aid, with assistance from others, not able to walk, or wheelchair-bound at all times), and whether patients recovered to their pre-fracture ambulation level. Psychosocial outcomes included post-operative living situation (i.e., living independently at home, living at home with assistance for activities of daily living, living with family or friends, or living in an institutional care facility), whether patients were able to have a meaningful conversation with others, and a 4-point Likert scale for pain experienced at the peak of recovery. Functional outcomes were assessed using the Katz ADL questionnaire for activities of daily living (ADL) [32,33]. Patients were asked about their level of independence (i.e., fully independent, help required from others or completely dependent) in the following categories: bathing, dressing, toileting, transferring in and out of a chair or wheelchair. Additionally, patients were asked if they were able to control their bladder and/or bowel movements, and if they were able to feed themselves (i.e., without assistance, help required from others, unable to feed themselves, or required tube feeding or parental nutrition). Missing values were excluded from analyses.

Descriptive statistics were used to report quantitative variables. Continuous variables were reported with median and interquartile ranges, and categorical variables with numbers and percentages. This was a purely descriptive study, and no comparison was made between groups. All statistical analyses were conducted using IBM SPSS Statistics™ for Windows, Version 28.0 (IBM Corp., 2021, Armonk, NY, USA). Data collection was carried out using Research Electronic Data Capture (REDCAP) version 14.0.27, an online Health Insurance Portability and Accountability Act (HIPAA)-compliant data management tool [34].

This study was registered with the Institutional Review Board (2019P003694), and was performed in accordance with the ethical standards laid down in the 1964 Declaration of Helsinki and its later amendments. This article was written in accordance with the Strengthening the Reporting of Observational Studies in Epidemiology (STROBE) guidelines for cross-sectional studies of the EQUATOR™ network [35].

3. Results

From a total of 426 patients treated for femur fractures, 87 were eligible for this study (Figure 1). After contacting eligible patients and/or their proxies to complete the survey, 37 patients participated and were included for analysis (42% response rate). Nine patients (24%) had died at the time of contact, so their proxies were asked to complete the survey in their stead. Reasons for eligible patients not participating in the study included not being willing to participate in the study or neither the patient nor proxy being able to be reached to complete the survey. Of all eligible patients, at least 25 patients had died at the start of the study, resulting in an overall mortality rate of 29%. The final cohort consisted of the 37 patients with outcomes collected either directly from the patient or their proxy.

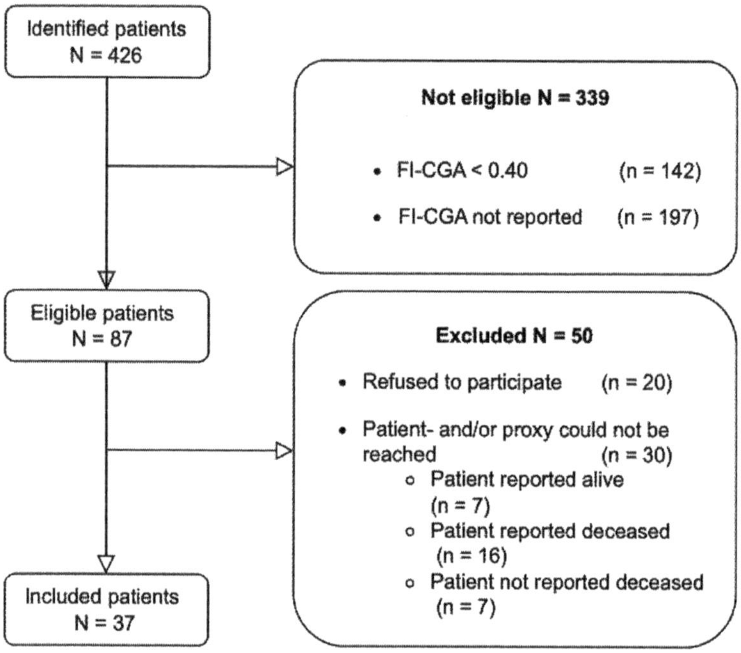

Figure 1. CONSORT Flow diagram of patient screening and inclusion.

Patient Demographics: At the time of injury, the median age was 85 years (IQR 78–92), with 70% of patients aged ≥80 (Table 1). Patients had a median FI-CGA of 0.48 (IQR 0.43–0.54) and were predominantly female (n = 28, 76%). Thirty-four patients were classified as high risk or very high risk, based upon the American Society of Anesthesiologists (ASA) score (ASA class ≥ III). Most patients (n = 29, 78%) presented with a proximal femur fracture, followed by six patients (16%) with a distal femur fracture, and two patients (5%) with a femoral shaft fracture.

Table 1. Patient characteristics (n = 37).

Patient Characteristics		N = 37 *
Age		85 (78–92)
Age ≥ 80		26 (70%)
Female		28 (76%)
ASA status	I	0 (0.0%)
	II	3 (8%)
	III	24 (65%)
	IV	10 (27%)
Frailty Index		0.48 (0.43–0.54)

Table 1. *Cont.*

Patient Characteristics	N = 37 *
Surgical information	
Type of fracture	
Proximal femur	29 (78%)
- Neck of femur	9
- Intertrochanteric	17
- Periprosthetic total hip	3
Shaft of femur	2 (5%)
Distal femur	6 (16%)
- Distal femur	5
- Periprosthetic total knee	1
Type of surgery	
Hip hemiarthroplasty	6 (16%)
Closed reduction and percutaneous pinning	1 (3%)
Intramedullary nail	16 (44%)
Dynamic hip screw	5 (14%)
Femur plating	5 (14%)
Revision total joint arthroplasty and/or femur plating	4 (8%)
Mortality	
Deceased at time of contact	9 (24%)

* Values are presented as median (inter quartile range) or number (n (%)).

Physical Function: Prior to injury, five patients (14%) were able to walk independently, twenty-nine patients (78%) could walk with walking aid(s) or a walker, and three patients (8%) were wheelchair-bound. At the best point in their recovery, one patient (3%) was able to walk independently, and twenty-five patients (69%) used walking aid(s) or a walker. Eleven patients (30%) were not able to walk at all or were wheelchair-bound, of whom five made use of a walker and three were already wheelchair-bound before injury. A total of eleven patients (30%) had recovered to the level of ambulation they had prior to their fracture (Figure 2). In terms of pain, twenty (54%) patients reported no to minimal pain, twelve patients (33%) still experienced mild to moderate pain, and three (8%) patients still experienced severe pain, although it is unclear if this pain related to their femur or other medical problems.

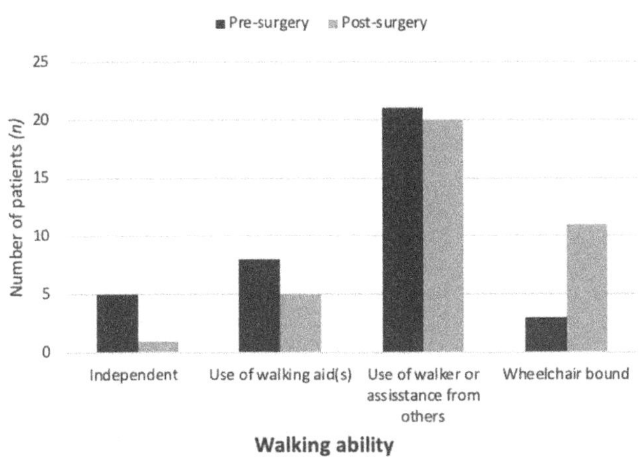

Distribution of ambulatory status pre- vs. post-surgery (n = 37)

Figure 2. Ambulatory status of severely frail patients before and after femur fracture fixation.

Psychosocial Outcomes: Prior to their femur fracture, seventeen patients (45%) lived at home, with or without assistance for ADL, seven (19%) patients lived with family or friends, and thirteen patients (35%) lived in an institutional care facility (Figure 3). At the best point in their recovery, six patients (16%) lived at home independently or with assistance for ADL, eleven patients (30%) lived with family or friends, and eighteen patients (49%) lived in an institutional care facility. Most patients (76%) reported that they were able to have a meaningful conversation with others.

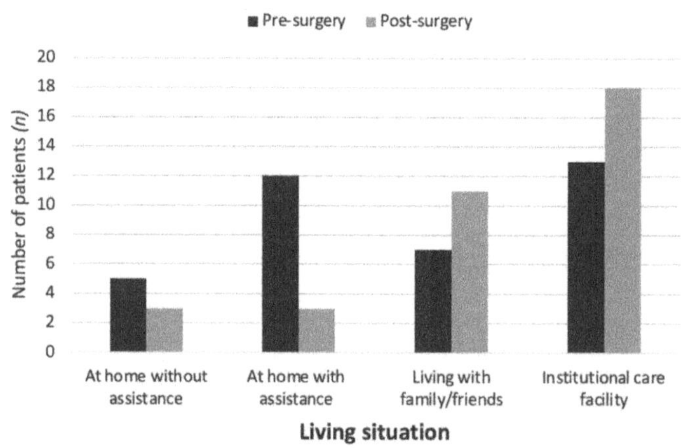

Distribution of living situation pre- vs. post-surgery (n = 37)

Figure 3. Living situation of severely frail patients before and after femur fracture fixation.

Activities of Daily Living: At the best point in their recovery, five (14%) patients were able to bathe themselves completely independent, twenty-five (69%) needed assistance with bathing, and six (17%) could only be washed in bed (Table 2). A total of thirty-one (84%) could dress themselves with or without assistance, and five (14%) were unable to dress themselves. Fourteen (39%) patients required no help from others when toileting, seventeen (47%) were able to go to the toilet with assistance from others, and five (14%) were unable to go to the toilet. Seventeen (47%) patients were able to transfer out of a (wheel)chair without assistance, while thirteen (36%) required help from others, and six (17%) were unable to transfer. Most patients were able to control their bladder and bowel movements (60%), and could eat without any assistance (78%), though five (14%) patients required tube feeding or parenteral nutrition.

Table 2. Activities of Daily Living (ADL) of severely frail patients at the best point in their recovery following femur fracture fixation.

ADL Domains	N = 36 * (%)
Bathing	
Without assistance	5 (14)
With assistance from others	25 (69)
Sponge bath required	6 (17)
Dressing	
Without assistance	9 (25)
With assistance from others	22 (61)
Completely dependent	5 (14)

Table 2. *Cont.*

ADL Domains	N = 36 * (%)
Toileting	
Without assistance	14 (39)
With assistance from others	17 (47)
Unable to go/use of urine bag	5 (14)
Transferring	
Without assistance	17 (47)
With assistance from others	13 (36)
Completely dependent	6 (17)
Bladder and/or bowel control	
In control	22 (61)
No control	14 (39)
Feeding	
Without assistance	28 (78)
With assistance from others	3 (8)
Completely dependent/tube- or parental nutrition	5 (14)

* Values are presented as number (n (%)); outcomes of ADL domains were missing for one patient.

4. Discussion

Femur fractures, particularly in the severely frail older adult population, represent a sentinel event in the decline towards the end of life, associated with a high degree of morbidity and mortality [3–5,9–11]. The prior literature has focused on post-operative complications and mortality, neglecting the long-term functional outcomes of these patients [25–27]. This cohort of 37 femoral fracture patients living with severe frailty, which mirrors Jones et al.'s distribution of frailty [18] and prior reported OGC care teams' target populations, demonstrates that while there is a high rate of 1-year mortality following surgical treatment of femur fractures, at the best point of recovery patients report overall positive outcomes in terms of freedom from pain, ambulatory ability, functional independence, and social interaction [5,11,27,36,37].

In terms of mobility, 30% of patients recovered to their previous ambulatory level, and 69% of patients were able to mobilize using a walking aid or walker in the 1-year following their injury. Functional independence varied per task and level of difficulty, with only 13% of patients able to bathe themselves independently, while almost 50% of patients were able to transfer from a chair. Various studies have reported on the loss of function and mobility in geriatric trauma patients [10,38–40], but none specifically captured the severely frail femur fracture population. For example, Magaziner et al. [38] reported that, among 536 hip fracture patients over 65 years older, nearly two-thirds of patients regained their pre-fracture walking ability, a little less than half of them had recovered physical activities of daily living, and just under one-third had a recovered IADL performance level. A Dutch prospective cohort study investigating the long-term ambulatory ability of previously ambulatory hip fracture patients aged above 65 years reported that 40% of patients remained ambulatory, but increasingly relied on assistive devices. Additionally, 12% of previous community ambulators transitioned to household ambulators, and 8% became non-functional ambulators [39]. Cooper et al. reported that, after 1-year, 60% of hip fracture patients lost independence in at least one essential activity of daily living (e.g., bathing or dressing themselves) [40]. These studies found significant loss of function and independence among older adults with femur fractures; however, they did not consider the impact of frailty on these outcomes, thus limiting the ability of clinicians to accurately predict severely frail patients' return to ambulation. The current study demonstrates that, even in the setting of severe frailty, the vast majority of patients report good freedom from pain and regain some ambulatory ability, even though for most there was a decline from their pre-injury level.

Psychosocially, over three-quarters of the studied patients were able to have a meaningful conversation, and the majority had minimal pain at the best point of their recovery.

Before their femur fracture, seventeen patients lived at home compared to six patients 1-year post-injury, indicating that eleven patients (30%) were institutionalized or needed to move in with family or friends after their injury. This finding is higher than the proportion of 10–20% reported in the general hip fracture population within Western industrialized countries [9], but in line with a smaller Dutch study showing that just over half of surviving patients returned to their original living circumstances 4-months following admission for a hip fracture [10]. In the severely frail patient population, sustaining a femur fracture is a life changing event, often leading to institutionalization and loss of independence, to some extent.

This study has several limitations. Given the target population, there was an expectedly low response rate of 42%, introducing a risk for non-response bias; however, the low response rate seen mirrors previously conducted patient- and/or proxy-reported survey studies among fracture patients, with response rates ranging between 38 and 66% [38,39,41–44]. Moreover, the response rate was impacted by the number of patients who had already died by the time of survey administration. We attempted to mitigate this limitation by including proxy-reported outcomes for patients who had died if proxies were reachable. The overall mortality rate of 29% among eligible patients highlights the substantial impact of femur fractures on the older frail trauma patient, and the challenges of studying long-term outcomes in this specific population. The presents study's subjective character and the reliance on retrospective observations of patients and proxies introduces the potential for recall bias. However, considering the current pitfalls in the field of geriatric trauma, where older frail patients are prone to selective loss to follow-up, selection bias, and survival bias [45], effort should be made to include these patients in clinical studies, including by proxy representation, as these patients might benefit most from the study's findings. Further, these patients are often on a declining medical trajectory, and it is difficult to ascribe their mortality and functional problems to their injury or surgery. Despite these limitations, this study is an important addition to the literature, and thus useful for clinicians with respect to shared decision-making, as it is the first and only study to examine and report on long-term patient-centered outcomes in severely frail femur fracture patients. To further validate current findings, future research should focus on extending follow-up to at least 2-years to better understand the long-term functional outcomes in this population. Moreover, this study made it evident that severely frail patients do achieve favorable functional outcomes after surgery, even with high mortality rates; this is, in a way, "hypothesis-forming". Future research studies are needed to explore the factors that contribute to poor and good recovery following femur fracture surgery, as well as appropriate treatment and intervention algorithms approaching these injuries in the frail population. Additionally, a previous investigation by our research team found a good correlation between patient- and proxy-reported pain interference and physical function in ambulatory, cognitively intact older patients [43], but it remains unknown how proxies' answers correlate with patients' psychosocial and functional outcomes. To better understand the use and value of proxy-reported measures, future research should investigate this relationship across other domains that apply to older adult and frail orthopedic trauma patients.

The primary focus of this study was to go 'beyond mortality', and it is the first study to gain insight in long-term functional and psychosocial outcomes of severely frail femur fracture patients. While femur fractures clearly represent a sentinel event for older adults, as both injury and its treatment are associated with a high risk of mortality, it is evident that a considerable share of patients regain the ability to ambulate with assistance, and report good pain relief. Despite some decline in their ability to live fully independently, many severely frail femur fracture patients continue to live with a certain degree of independence. This information can help treating physicians and surgeons to better counsel patients and their loved ones during shared decision-making conversations by informing them of what to expect functionally following surgery for femur fractures in the severely frail population. In this patient-centered approach, alignment of treatment and goals of care may improve quality of life and patient/proxy satisfaction with care. Further research is needed to investigate the factors that impact patient- and proxy-reported outcomes in this patient population, as well as the additional recourses needed to care for this patient population, to facilitate better alignment of treatment decisions and patient goals of care.

Author Contributions: Conceptualization, H.J.S., L.C., H.J. and M.J.W.; methodology, all authors; software N.H.M.P. and J.H.R.; investigation and data curation, N.H.M.P., J.H.R., D.T.B., A.S. and H.J.S.; validation and formal analysis, all authors; resources, N.H.M.P., J.H.R., D.T.B. and H.J.S.; writing—original draft preparation, N.H.M.P., J.H.R., D.T.B. and H.J.S.; writing—review and editing, all authors; supervision, L.C., H.J. and M.J.W. All authors have read and agreed to the published version of the manuscript.

Funding: This research received no external funding.

Institutional Review Board Statement: The study was conducted in accordance with the Declaration of Helsinki, and was approved by the Institutional Review Board of Mass General Brigham (2019P003694, 19 February 2020).

Informed Consent Statement: Informed consent was obtained from all subjects involved in the study.

Data Availability Statement: The data presented in this study are available on request from the corresponding authors. The data are not publicly available due to legal restrictions.

Conflicts of Interest: The authors declare no conflicts of interest.

References

1. Christensen, K.; Doblhammer, G.; Rau, R.; Vaupel, J.W. Ageing Populations: The Challenges Ahead. *Lancet* **2009**, *374*, 1196–1208. [CrossRef]
2. Manton, K.G. Recent Declines in Chronic Disability in the Elderly U.S. Population: Risk Factors and Future Dynamics. *Proc. Annu. Rev. Public Health* **2008**, *29*, 91–113. [CrossRef]
3. Clegg, A.; Young, J.; Iliffe, S.; Rikkert, M.O.; Rockwood, K. Frailty in Elderly People. *Lancet* **2013**, *381*, 752–762. [CrossRef]
4. Zhao, F.; Tang, B.; Hu, C.; Wang, B.; Wang, Y.; Zhang, L. The Impact of Frailty on Posttraumatic Outcomes in Older Trauma Patients: A Systematic Review and Meta-Analysis. *J. Trauma Acute Care Surg.* **2020**, *88*, 546–554. [CrossRef]
5. Merino-Rueda, L.R.; Rubio-Sáez, I.; Mills, S.; Rubio-Suárez, J.C. Mortality after Distal Femur Fractures in the Elderly. *Injury* **2021**, *52*, S71–S75. [CrossRef]
6. Pilotto, A.; Custodero, C.; Maggi, S.; Polidori, M.C.; Veronese, N.; Ferrucci, L. A Multidimensional Approach to Frailty in Older People. *Ageing Res. Rev.* **2020**, *60*, 101047. [CrossRef]
7. Cohen, C.I.; Benyaminov, R.; Rahman, M.; Ngu, D.; Reinhardt, M. Frailty: A Multidimensional Biopsychosocial Syndrome. *Med. Clin. N. Am.* **2023**, *107*, 183–197. [CrossRef]
8. Eagles, D.; Godwin, B.; Cheng, W.; Moors, J.; Figueira, S.; Khoury, L.; Fournier, K.; Lampron, J. A Systematic Review and Meta-Analysis Evaluating Geriatric Consultation on Older Trauma Patients. *J. Trauma Acute Care Surg.* **2020**, *88*, 446–453. [CrossRef]
9. Dyer, S.M.; Crotty, M.; Fairhall, N.; Magaziner, J.; Beaupre, L.A.; Cameron, I.D.; Sherrington, C. A Critical Review of the Long-Term Disability Outcomes Following Hip Fracture. *BMC Geriatr.* **2016**, *16*, 158. [CrossRef]
10. Van Balen, R.; Steyerberg, E.W.; Polder, J.J.; Ribbers, T.L.M.; Habbema, J.D.F.; Cools, H.J.M. Hip Fracture in Elderly Patients Outcomes for Function, Quality of Life, and Type of Residence. *Clin. Orthop. Relat. Res.* **1996**, *390*, 232–243. [CrossRef]
11. Grigoryan, K.V.; Javedan, H.; Rudolph, J.L. Orthogeriatric Care Models and Outcomes in Hip Fracture Patients: A Systematic Review and Meta-Analysis. *J. Orthop. Trauma* **2013**, *28*, e49–e55. [CrossRef]
12. Uzoigwe, C.E.; Burnand, H.G.F.; Cheesman, C.L.; Aghedo, D.O.; Faizi, M.; Middleton, R.G. Early and Ultra-Early Surgery in Hip Fracture Patients Improves Survival. *Injury* **2013**, *44*, 726–729. [CrossRef]
13. Simunovic, N.; Devereaux, P.J.; Sprague, S.; Guyatt, G.H.; Schemitsch, E.; DeBeer, J.; Bhandari, M. Effect of Early Surgery after Hip Fracture on Mortality and Complications: Systematic Review and Meta-Analysis. *CMAJ Can. Med. Assoc. J.* **2010**, *182*, 1609–1616. [CrossRef]
14. Marcantonio, E.R.; Flacker, J.M.; Michaels, M.; Resnick, N.M. Delirium Is Independently Associated with Poor Functional Recovery after Hip Fracture. *J. Am. Geriatr. Soc.* **2000**, *48*, 618–624. [CrossRef]
15. Cole, E. Open Access Scandinavian Journal of Trauma, Resuscitation and Emergency Medicine. *Scand. J. Trauma Resusc. Emerg. Med.* **2024**, *32*, 1. [CrossRef]
16. Chen, P.; Hung, W.W. Geriatric Orthopedic Co-Management of Older Adults with Hip Fracture: An Emerging Standard. *Ann. Transl. Med.* **2015**, *3*, 224. [CrossRef] [PubMed]
17. Jones, D.M.; Song, X.; Rockwood, K. Operationalizing a Frailty Index from a Standardized Comprehensive Geriatric Assessment. *J. Am. Geriatr. Soc.* **2004**, *52*, 1929–1933. [CrossRef]

18. Jones, D.; Song, X.; Mitnitski, A.; Rockwood, K. Evaluation of a Frailty Index Based on a Comprehensive Geriatric Assessment in a Population Based Study of Elderly Canadians. *Aging Clin. Exp. Res.* **2005**, *17*, 465–471. [CrossRef]
19. Cooper, L.; Loewenthal, J.; Frain, L.N.; Tulebaev, S.; Cardin, K.; Hshieh, T.T.; Dumontier, C.; Streiter, S.; Joseph, C.; Hilt, A.; et al. From Research to Bedside: Incorporation of a CGA-Based Frailty Index among Multiple Comanagement Services. *J. Am. Geriatr. Soc.* **2022**, *70*, 90–98. [CrossRef]
20. Mitnitski, A.B.; Mogilner, A.J.; Rockwood, K. Accumulation of Deficits as a Proxy Measure of Aging. *Sci. World J.* **2001**, *1*, 323–336. [CrossRef]
21. McDermid, R.C.; Stelfox, H.T.; Bagshaw, S.M. Frailty in the Critically Ill: A Novel Concept. *Crit. Care* **2011**, *15*, 301. [CrossRef] [PubMed]
22. Muscedere, J.; Waters, B.; Varambally, A.; Bagshaw, S.M.; Boyd, J.G.; Maslove, D.; Sibley, S.; Rockwood, K. The Impact of Frailty on Intensive Care Unit Outcomes: A Systematic Review and Meta-Analysis. *Intensive Care Med.* **2017**, *43*, 1105–1122. [CrossRef] [PubMed]
23. Ritt, M.; Rádi, K.H.; Schwarz, C.; Bollheimer, L.C.; Sieber, C.C.; Gassmann, K.G. A Comparison of Frailty Indexes Based on a Comprehensive Geriatric Assessment for the Prediction of Adverse Outcomes. *J. Nutr. Health Aging* **2007**, *20*, 760–767. [CrossRef] [PubMed]
24. Rockwood, K.; Song, X.; Mitnitski, A. Changes in Relative Fitness and Frailty across the Adult Lifespan: Evidence from the Canadian National Population Health Survey. *Can. Med. Assoc. J.* **2011**, *183*, 487–494. [CrossRef] [PubMed]
25. Lefaivre, K.A.; Macadam, S.A.; Davidson, D.J.; Gandhi, R.; Chan, H.; Broekhuyse, H.M.; Epi, S.M. Length of Stay, Mortality, Morbidity and Delay to Surgery in Hip Fractures. *Bone Jt. J.* **2009**, *91*, 922–927.
26. Katsoulis, M.; Benetou, V.; Karapetyan, T.; Feskanich, D.; Grodstein, F.; Pettersson-Kymmer, U.; Eriksson, S.; Wilsgaard, T.; Jørgensen, L.; Ahmed, L.A.; et al. Excess Mortality after Hip Fracture in Elderly Persons from Europe and the USA: The CHANCES Project. *J. Intern. Med.* **2017**, *281*, 300–310. [CrossRef] [PubMed]
27. Menéndez-Colino, R.; Alarcon, T.; Gotor, P.; Queipo, R.; Ramírez-Martín, R.; Otero, A.; González-Montalvo, J.I. Baseline and Pre-Operative 1-Year Mortality Risk Factors in a Cohort of 509 Hip Fracture Patients Consecutively Admitted to a Co-Managed Orthogeriatric Unit (FONDA Cohort). *Injury* **2018**, *49*, 656–661. [CrossRef] [PubMed]
28. Roth, T.; Kammerlander, C.; Gosch, M.; Luger, T.J.; Blauth, M. Outcome in Geriatric Fracture Patients and How It Can Be Improved. *Osteoporos. Int.* **2010**, *21*, 615–619. [CrossRef]
29. AO Foundation. *AO/OTA Fracture and Dislocation Classification. Introduction to the Classification of Long-Bone Fractures*; AO Foundation: Davos, Switzerland, 2018.
30. AO Foundation. Unified Classification System for Periprosthetic Fractures (UCPF). *J. Orthop. Trauma* **2018**, *32*, S141–S144. [CrossRef]
31. World Health Organization. *International Statistical Classification of Diseases and Related Health Problems*, 10th ed.; World Health Organization: Geneva, Switzerland, 2023. Available online: https://www.icd10data.com (accessed on 25 February 2024).
32. Katz, S.; Ford, A.; Moskowitz, R.; Jackson, B.; Jaffe, M. Studies of Illness in the Aged: The Index of Adl: A Standardized Measure of Biological and Psychosocial Function. *JAMA* **1963**, *185*, 914–919. [CrossRef]
33. Edemekong, P.F.; Bomgaars, D.; Sukumaran, S.; Levy, S.B. Activities of Daily Living. In *StatPearls*; StatPearls Publishing: Treasure Island, FL, USA, 2019.
34. Harris, P.A.; Taylor, R.; Thielke, R.; Payne, J.; Gonzalez, N.; Conde, J.G. Research Electronic Data Capture (REDCap)-A Metadata Driven Methodology and Workflow Process for Providing Translational Research Informatics Support. *J. Biomed. Inf.* **2008**, *42*, 377–381. [CrossRef] [PubMed]
35. von Elm, E.; Altman, D.; Egger, M.; Pocock, S.; Gotzsche, P.; Vandenbroucke, J. Annals of Internal Medicine Academia and Clinic The Strengthening the Reporting of Observational Studies in Epidemiology (STROBE) Statement: Guidelines for Reporting. *Ann. Intern. Med.* **2007**, *147*, 573–577. [CrossRef] [PubMed]
36. Baroni, M.; Serra, R.; Boccardi, V.; Ercolani, S.; Zengarini, E.; Casucci, P.; Valecchi, R.; Rinonapoli, G.; Caraffa, A.; Mecocci, P.; et al. The Orthogeriatric Comanagement Improves Clinical Outcomes of Hip Fracture in Older Adults. *Osteoporos. Int.* **2019**, *30*, 907–916. [CrossRef] [PubMed]
37. Alizai, Q.; Colosimo, C.; Hosseinpour, H.; Stewart, C.; Bhogadi, S.K.; Nelson, A.; Spencer, A.L.; Ditillo, M.; Magnotti, L.J.; Joseph, B. It's Not All Black and White: The Effect of Increasing Severity of Frailty on Outcomes of Geriatric Trauma Patients. *J. Trauma Acute Care Surg.* **2023**, *96*, 434–442. [CrossRef] [PubMed]
38. Magaziner, J.; Simonsick, E.M.; Kashner, T.M.; Hebel, J.R.; Kenzora, J.E. Predictors of Functional Recovery One Year Following Hospital Discharge for Hip Fracture: A Prospective Study. *J. Gerontol.* **1990**, *45*, M101–M107. [CrossRef] [PubMed]
39. Koval, K.J.; Skovron, M.L.; Aharonoff, G.B.; Meadows, S.E.; Zuckerman, J.D. Ambulatory Ability after Hip Fracture A Prospective Study in Geriatric Patients. *Clin. Orthop. Relat. Res.* **1995**, *310*, 150–159.
40. Cooper, C.; Cummings, S.; Lyons, A.; Karpf, D.B.; Tamayo-Orozco, J.; Black, D.; Ross, P.D.; Johnell, O. The Crippling Consequences of Fractures and Their Impact on Quality of Life. *Am. J. Med.* **1997**, *103*, S12–S19. [CrossRef] [PubMed]
41. Turner, N.; Dinh, J.M.; Durham, J.; Schroder, L.K.; Ziegenfuss, J.Y.; Switzer, J.A. Development of a Questionnaire to Assess Patient Priorities in Hip Fracture Care. *Geriatr. Orthop. Surg. Rehabil.* **2020**, *11*, 1–10. [CrossRef]

42. Dvorzhinskiy, A.; Gausden, E.B.; Levack, A.E.; Nwachukwu, B.U.; Nguyen, J.; Gadinsky, N.E.; Wellman, D.S.; Lorich, D.G. The Performance of PROMIS Computer Adaptive Testing for Patient-Reported Outcomes in Hip Fracture Surgery: A Pilot Study. *Arch. Orthop. Trauma Surg.* **2022**, *142*, 417–424. [CrossRef]
43. Alvarez-Nebreda, M.L.; Heng, M.; Rosner, B.; McTague, M.; Javedan, H.; Harris, M.B.; Weaver, M.J. Reliability of Proxy-Reported Patient-Reported Outcomes Measurement Information System Physical Function and Pain Interference Responses for Elderly Patients with Musculoskeletal Injury. *J. Am. Acad. Orthop. Surg.* **2019**, *27*, E156–E165. [CrossRef]
44. Nijdam, T.M.P.; Laane, D.W.P.M.; Schiepers, T.E.E.; Smeeing, D.P.J.; Kempen, D.H.R.; Willems, H.C.; van der Velde, D. The Goals of Care in Acute Setting for Geriatric Patients in Case of a Hip Fracture. *Eur. J. Trauma Emerg. Surg.* **2023**, *49*, 1835–1844. [CrossRef] [PubMed]
45. O'hara, N.N.; Degani, Y.; Marvel, D.; Wells, D.; Mullins, C.D.; Wegener, S.; Frey, K.; Joseph, T.; Hurst, J.; Castillo, R.; et al. Which Orthopaedic Trauma Patients Are Likely to Refuse to Participate in a Clinical Trial? A Latent Class Analysis on Behalf of PREVENT CLOT Stakeholder Committee. *BMJ Open* **2019**, *9*, e032631. [CrossRef] [PubMed]

Journal of
Clinical Medicine

MDPI

Article

Rehabilitation of Frail Older Adults after Hip Fracture Surgery: Predictors for the Length of Geriatric Rehabilitation Stay at a Skilled Nursing Home

Sanne M. Krakers [1,2,*,†], Sanne Woudsma [3,†], Dieuwke van Dartel [1,2], Marloes Vermeer [4], Miriam M. R. Vollenbroek-Hutten [2], Johannes H. Hegeman [1,2] and on behalf of the Up&Go after a Hip Fracture Group [‡]

1 Department of Trauma Surgery, Ziekenhuisgroep Twente, 7609 PP Almelo, The Netherlands
2 Department of Biomedical Signals and Systems, University of Twente, 7500 AE Enschede, The Netherlands
3 Geriatric Rehabilitation Department, ZorgAccent, 7442 KH Nijverdal, The Netherlands
4 ZGT Academy, Ziekenhuisgroep Twente, 7609 PP Almelo, The Netherlands
* Correspondence: s.m.krakers@utwente.nl
† These authors contributed equally to this work.
‡ Collaborators of the Up&Go after a Hip Fracture Group is provided in the Acknowledgements.

Abstract: Background: Approximately 50% of older patients hospitalized for hip fractures are admitted to a geriatric rehabilitation department at a skilled nursing home. Given the wide variation in rehabilitation stay lengths, predicting the length of stay upon hospital discharge would help manage patients' recovery expectations and create appropriate therapy schedules. Existing literature on length of stay predictors included both acute hospital and in-hospital rehabilitation phases or involved small sample sizes. The present study aims to identify predictors for the length of geriatric rehabilitation stay in skilled nursing homes for older patients after hip fracture surgery upon hospital discharge. **Methods:** This retrospective cohort study was conducted from 1 October 2017 to 1 July 2023, including 561 patients. Potential predictors of the length of geriatric rehabilitation stay were first tested univariately, with variables showing $p < 0.15$ entered into a multivariate forward linear regression model. **Results:** This model identified the following independent predictors of a longer length of geriatric rehabilitation stay: Functional Ambulation Categories (FACs) 0 (B = 29.9, 95% CI 24.1–35.7), 1 (B = 18.0, 95% CI 11.8–24.2), 2 (B = 12.0, 95% CI 7.1–17.0), or 3 (B = 3.6, 95% CI −1.2–9.4) at hospital discharge vs. FAC 4, living independently with home care services (B = 5.9, 95% CI 2.5–9.3) or in a residential home prior to the hip fracture (B = 0.2, 95% CI −7.4–7.8) vs. living independently without home care services, non- or partial weight-bearing mobilization vs. full weight-bearing mobilization (B = 15.4, 95% CI 8.5–22.2), internal fixation vs. hemiarthroplasty (B = 4.7, 95% CI 1.4–7.9), in-hospital delirium (B = 7.0, 95% CI 2.2–11.7), and in-hospital heart failure (B = 7.9, 95% CI 0.5–15.3). The explained variance was 32.0%. **Conclusions:** This study identified FAC at hospital discharge, premorbid living situation, postoperative weight-bearing protocol, surgery type, in-hospital delirium, and in-hospital heart failure as independent predictors of the length of geriatric rehabilitation stay. Future investigations are needed to identify additional predictors, such as cognitive functioning, to better predict the length of geriatric rehabilitation stay upon hospital discharge.

Keywords: geriatric rehabilitation; hip fracture; length of stay; surgery; older patients; predictors

1. Introduction

After hip fracture surgery, approximately 50% of patients aged ≥70 years are admitted to a geriatric rehabilitation department at a skilled nursing home [1]. In 2017, the Department of Trauma Surgery at Ziekenhuisgroep Twente (ZGT), Almelo, the Netherlands, developed and implemented a multidisciplinary transmural care pathway in collaboration with three skilled nursing homes (TriviumMeulenbeltZorg, ZorgAccent, and Carintreggeland) in the vicinity of ZGT to synchronize the care processes and to gain more insights into the rehabilitation process of older patients after hip fracture surgery. In all skilled nursing homes, there was a "rehabilitation climate", meaning that every daily activity was used as a therapeutic moment. Both caregivers and family members actively participated in the rehabilitation process. Multidisciplinary treatment was focused on the patient's rehabilitation goals. The multidisciplinary team consisted of a nursing home physician, physiotherapist, occupational therapist, dietician, psychologist, and the nursing staff. For all geriatric rehabilitation departments, the received therapy by the physiotherapist was the same. However, the first results of the multidisciplinary transmural care pathway showed an interquartile range (IQR) of 25–50 days for the length of geriatric rehabilitation stay among patients [2].

Due to the wide variation in the length of stay in the geriatric rehabilitation facility, it is difficult for hospital healthcare professionals to prepare patients for what to expect during the rehabilitation period and for geriatric rehabilitation healthcare professionals to create appropriate therapy schedules. It is desirable to be able to predict the length of geriatric rehabilitation stay upon hospital discharge. This enables patients to manage their recovery expectations at the rehabilitation department of a skilled nursing home. Being aware of what to expect helps patients prepare for what is coming and set realistic goals. Furthermore, predicting the length of geriatric rehabilitation stay upon hospital discharge may help healthcare professionals identify the rehabilitation needs of each patient. For example, patients who are expected to recover rapidly may benefit from a more intensive therapy schedule, allowing for the most efficient organization of rehabilitation therapy.

There is a great diversity in the literature concerning factors influencing the length of geriatric rehabilitation stay in older patients after hip fracture surgery [3–5]. Higher age, trochanteric and subtrochanteric fractures compared to intracapsular fractures, comorbidities (Parkinson's disease, diabetes, and dementia), complications (wound infection, delirium, urinary tract infection, and pneumonia), independent gait at hospital discharge compared to dependent gait, living alone prior to the hip fracture compared to living together, using mobility aids prior to the hip fracture compared to being mobile without aids, and a lower Barthel score at geriatric rehabilitation admission were found as predictors for a longer length of geriatric rehabilitation stay [3–5]. However, these variables were found in studies with small sample sizes, were collected during both the hospital and rehabilitation phases, or were associated with the total length of hospital stay, including the acute hospital and in-hospital rehabilitation phases. It therefore remains unclear which factors influence the actual length of geriatric rehabilitation stay at a skilled nursing home upon discharge from the hospital. This lack of clarity currently renders predictions of the length of geriatric rehabilitation stay upon hospital discharge impossible.

The aim of this study is to identify predictors for the length of geriatric rehabilitation stay at a skilled nursing home for older patients after hip fracture surgery upon hospital discharge, using data collected from the transmural care pathway.

2. Materials and Methods

2.1. Study Design

A retrospective cohort study was conducted from the first of October 2017 until the first of July 2023. Inclusion criteria for the study were patients aged ≥70 years who underwent hip fracture surgery (hemiarthroplasty or internal fixation) at the Department of Trauma Surgery at ZGT and rehabilitated at one of the three participating skilled nursing homes (TriviumMeulenbeltZorg, ZorgAccent, and Carintreggeland) (Figure 1). Exclusion criteria for this study were pathological or periprosthetic fractures or incomplete data collection of the rehabilitation process.

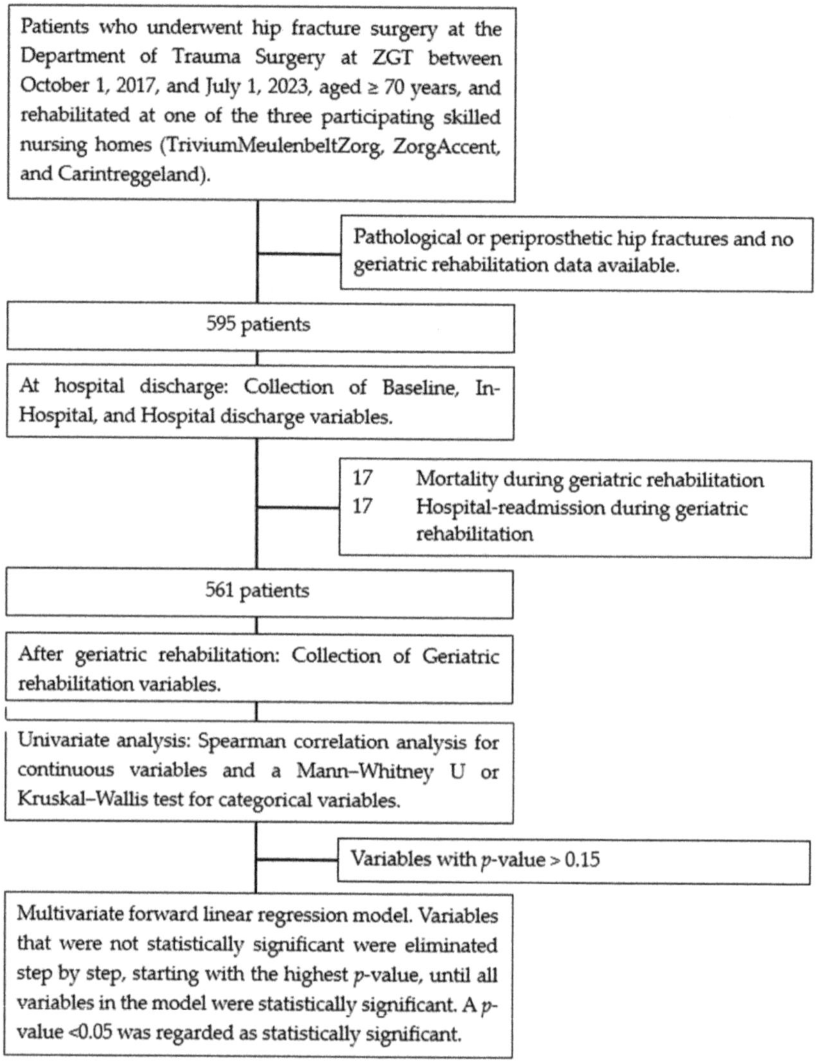

Figure 1. Flowchart of study design.

The Medical Ethical Committee of Twente stated that this study did not require an assessment by the Medical Ethical Committee according to Dutch law. The study was approved by the Institutional Review Board of ZGT. All patients gave written informed consent to participate.

The primary outcome was the length of geriatric rehabilitation stay at the skilled nursing homes in days. For this study, baseline, in-hospital, hospital discharge, and geriatric rehabilitation variables were collected from the transmural care pathway database. Data were entered into Castor EDC, a cloud-based Electronic Data Capture platform (ISO 27001 certified) [6].

2.2. Baseline Variables

Age, gender, premorbid living situation, living alone versus together, availability of non-professional help, need for climbing stairs, Pre-Fracture Mobility Score (PFMS), premorbid Katz Index of Independence in Activities of Daily Living (Katz-ADL6), Charlson Comorbidity Index (CCI), American Society of Anesthesiologists physical status classification (ASA score), and Short Nutritional Assessment Questionnaire (SNAQ) were collected as baseline variables.

The (P)FMS assesses the patients' independence in walking and ranges from 1 (freely mobile without aids) to 5 (no functional mobility) [7]. The Katz-ADL6 assesses patients' independence in ADL, where a score of 0 means fully independent in ADL and a score of 6 means fully dependent in ADL [8]. The CCI measures comorbidity, where a higher score means a higher comorbidity burden [9]. The ASA score measures the condition of a patient prior to surgery, with ASA 1–2 for a patient who has no or mild systematic diseases, ASA 3–4 for a patient who has severe systematic diseases, and ASA 5 for a moribund patient [10]. The SNAQ is a malnutrition screening tool, with SNAQ ≥ 2 indicating moderately malnourished patients and SNAQ ≥ 3 severely malnourished patients [11].

2.3. In-Hospital Variables

Hemoglobin (Hb) at hospital admission, hip fracture type, time until surgery, surgical treatment, postoperative weight-bearing protocol, and in-hospital complications were collected as in-hospital variables.

2.4. Hospital Discharge Variables

Functional Ambulation Categories (FACs) at hospital discharge, Fracture Mobility Score (FMS) at hospital discharge, Katz-ADL6 at hospital discharge, admission to which skilled nursing home (TriviumMeulenbeltZorg, Carintreggeland, or ZorgAccent), and the length of hospital stay were collected as hospital discharge variables.

The FAC assesses the patients' independence in walking and ranges from 0 (no functional mobility) to 5 (fully independent mobility) [7].

2.5. Geriatric Rehabilitation Variables

The hospital readmission rate and mortality rate were recorded as geriatric rehabilitation variables. The length of hospital might be influenced by logistical factors that cannot be predicted or influenced and, therefore, was excluded as a potential predictor of the primary outcome measure.

2.6. Statistical Analysis

Continuous data were described as mean with standard deviation (SD) or as median with interquartile range (IQR) in case of a skewed distribution. Categorical data were presented as numbers with the corresponding percentage. Relationships between baseline, in-hospital, and hospital discharge variables and length of geriatric rehabilitation stay were first tested univariately using a Pearson or Spearman correlation analysis for continuous variables and an independent t-test, Mann–Whitney U test, ANOVA, or Kruskal–Wallis test for categorical variables. Variables with a p-value < 0.15 were entered into a multivariate forward linear regression model to ensure that no potential variables would be missed. Subsequently, variables that were not statistically significant were eliminated step by step, starting with the highest p-value, until all variables in the model were statistically significant. A p-value < 0.05 was regarded as statistically significant. All analyses were performed using SPSS version 22.0 (IBM Corp., Armonk, NY, USA).

3. Results

In the study period from the first of October 2017 until the first of July 2023, a total of 604 older patients were included. Of those patients, 9 had incomplete data (no geriatric rehabilitation data available) and were excluded, leaving 595 older patients in this study (Table 1).

Table 1. Patient characteristics.

		Total (*n* = 595)
Baseline variables		
Age in years; mean (SD)		82.5 (7.8)
Female gender; *n* (%)		422 (70.9)
Premorbid living situation; *n* (%)	Independent without home care services Independent with home care services Residential home	365 (59.8) 207 (34.8) 29 (4.9)
Living together; *n* (%)		198 (38.3)
Availability non-professional help; *n* (%)		509 (85.5)
Need for climbing stairs; *n* (%)		155 (26.1)
PFMS; *n* (%)	1—Freely mobile without aids 2—Mobile outdoors with one aid 3—Mobile outdoors with two aids or frame 4—Some indoor mobility but never goes outside without help 5—No functional mobility	228 (38.3) 60 (10.1) 264 (44.4) 37 (6.2) 0 (0)
Premorbid Katz-ADL6; median (IQR)		0 (0–2)
CCI; median (IQR)		1 (0–2)
ASA score; *n* (%)	ASA 1–2 ASA 3–4 ASA 5	184 (30.9) 406 (68.2) 0 (0.0)
SNAQ; median (IQR)		0 (0–0)
In-hospital variables		
Hb at hospital admission; median (IQR)		8.5 (7.0–9.0)
Hip fracture type; *n* (%)	Femoral neck Trochanteric/subtrochanteric femur	299 (50.3) 296 (49.7)
Time until surgery; *n* (%)	0–24 h 24–36 h 36–48 h > 48 h	358 (60.2) 139 (23.4) 58 (9.7) 40 (6.7)
Surgical treatment; *n* (%)	Internal fixation: PFNA, DHS, cannulated screws Hemiarthroplasty	356 (59.8) 239 (40.2)
Postoperative weight-bearing protocol; *n* (%)	Full weight-bearing Partial/non-weight-bearing	558 (93.8) 37 (6.2)
In-hospital complications; *n* (%)	Anemia Heart failure Delirium Pneumonia Pressure ulcers Urinary tract infection Wound infection Uncomplicated	120 (20.2) 28 (4.6) 74 (12.4) 57 (9.6) 29 (4.9) 36 (6.1) 3 (0.5) 282 (47.4)
Hospital discharge variables		
FACs at hospital discharge; *n* (%)	0—No functional mobility 1—Dependent in mobility level 2 2—Dependent in mobility level 1 3—Independent mobility under supervision 4—Independent mobility on a flat surface	93 (15.6) 67 (11.3) 167 (28.1) 176 (29.6) 90 (15.1)

Table 1. *Cont.*

FMS at hospital discharge; *n* (%)	1—Freely mobile without aids	0 (0)
	2—Mobile outdoors with one aid	0 (0)
	3—Mobile outdoors with two aids or frame	28 (4.7)
	4—Some indoor mobility but never goes outside without help	462 (77.6)
	5—No functional mobility	105 (17.6)
Katz-ADL6 at hospital discharge; median (IQR)		4 (4–5)
Rehabilitation department skilled nursing home; *n* (%)	Skilled nursing home A	304 (51.1)
	Skilled nursing home B	215 (36.1)
	Skilled nursing home C	76 (12.8)
Length of hospital stay in days; median (IQR)		8 (6–10)
Geriatric rehabilitation variables		
Hospital-readmission during rehabilitation; *n* (%)		17 (2.9)
Mortality during rehabilitation; *n* (%)		17 (2.9)
Length of geriatric rehabilitation stay in days; median (IQR)		35 (24–47)

SD, standard deviation; n, number; (P)FMS, (Pre-)Fracture Mobility Score; Katz-ADL, Katz Index of Independence in Activities of Daily Living; IQR, interquartile range; CCI, Charlson Comorbidity Index; ASA, American Society of Anesthesiologists physical status classification; SNAQ, Short Nutritional Assessment Questionnaire; Hb, hemoglobin; PFNA, Proximal Femoral Nail Antirotation; DHS, Dynamic Hip Screw; FACs, Functional Ambulation Categories.

3.1. Patient Characteristics

The mean (SD) age was 82.5 (7.8) years and 70.9% (n = 422) of the patients were female. Severe comorbidities (ASA $\geq$ 3) were observed in 68.2% (n = 406) of the patients. In 50.3% (n = 299), the hip fracture type was a femoral neck fracture and in 49.7% (n = 296), a trochanteric or subtrochanteric femur fracture. In 60.2% (n = 358) of the patients, the time until surgery was within 24 h and in 6.7% (n = 40) after 48 h. In 59.8% (n = 356), the surgical treatment was internal fixation (Proximal Femur Nail Antirotation (PFNA), Dynamic Hip Screw (DHS), or cannulated screws) and in 40.2% (n = 239), a hemiarthroplasty. After surgical treatment, 93.8% (n = 558) of the patients were allowed to put full weight on the operated leg. During the hospital stay, 47.4% (n = 282) of the patients had no complications, 20.2% (n = 120) were anemic and needed a blood transfusion, 12.4% (n = 74) had delirium, and 4.6% (n = 28) heart failure.

3.2. Living Situation and Functional Status

Prior to the hip fracture, 59.8% (n = 356) of the patients were living independently without home care services, 34.8% (n = 207) independently with home care services, and 4.9% (n = 29) were living in a residential home. Furthermore, 33.3% (n = 198) of the patients were living together with a relative and 85.5% (n = 509) could invoke non-professional help. Before the fracture, 38.3% (n = 228) of the patients were able to walk fully independently without aids (PFMS 1), 54.5% (n = 324) used a walking aid (PFMS 2) or aids (PFMS 3), and 6.2% (n = 37) were only able to walk independently indoors (PFMS 4). Most patients were independent in ADL before the fracture (median (IQR) premorbid Katz-ADL6 was 0 (0–2)). At hospital discharge, 15.6% (n = 93) of the older patients had no functional mobility (FAC 0), 69.0% (n = 410) needed assistance during walking (FAC 1–3), and 15.1% (n = 90) were independent in mobility (FAC 4–5). In addition, most patients were dependent in ADL at hospital discharge (median (IQR) Katz-ADL6 was 4 (4–5)).

3.3. Length of Hospital and Geriatric Rehabilitation Stay

The median (IQR) length of hospital stay was 8 (6–10) days. The median (IQR) length of geriatric rehabilitation stay at the skilled nursing home was 35 (24–47) days.

Furthermore, 17 (2.9%) patients died during the rehabilitation phase and 17 (2.9%) patients were readmitted to the hospital during geriatric rehabilitation stay.

3.4. Predictors for Length of Geriatric Rehabilitation Stay

For the univariate analysis, 34 (5.7%) patients were excluded, because of readmission to the hospital or death during a geriatric rehabilitation stay. Results from the univariate analysis are presented in Table 2.

Table 2. Univariate analysis and multivariate linear regression analysis factors length of geriatric rehabilitation stay.

		Univariate Analysis * (n = 561)	Multivariate Linear Regression Analysis (n = 561)	
		p	B (95% CI)	p
Baseline variables				
Age		0.020		
Female gender		0.713		
Premorbid living situation	Independent without home care services Independent with home care services Residential home	<0.001	ref. 5.9 (2.5–9.3) 0.2 (−7.4–7.8)	<0.001 0.952
Living together		0.267		
Availability non-professional help		0.501		
Need for climbing stairs		0.127		
PFMS	1—Freely mobile without aids 2—Mobile outdoors with one aid 3—Mobile outdoors with two aids or frame 4—Some indoor mobility but never goes outside without help 5—No functional mobility	<0.001		
Premorbid Katz-ADL6		<0.001		
CCI		0.871		
ASA score	ASA 1–2 ASA 3–4	0.003		
SNAQ		0.983		
In-hospital variables				
Hb hospital admission		0.667		
Hip fracture type	Femoral neck Trochanteric/subtrochanteric femur	0.025		
Time until surgery	0–24 h 24–36 h 36–48 h >48 h	0.405		
Surgical treatment	Internal fixation: PFNA, DHS, cannulated screws Hemiarthroplasty	<0.001	4.7 (1.4–7.9) ref.	0.005
Postoperative weight-bearing protocol	Full weight-bearing Partial/non-weight-bearing	<0.001	ref. 15.4 (8.5–22.2)	<0.001

Table 2. *Cont.*

In-hospital complications	Anemia	0.008		
	Heart failure	0.020	7.9 (0.5–15.3)	0.037
	Delirium	<0.001	7.0 (2.2–11.7)	0.004
	Pneumonia	0.871		
	Pressure ulcers	0.268		
	Urinary tract infection	0.348		
	Wound infection	0.260		
	Uncomplicated	<0.001		
Hospital discharge variables				
FAC at hospital discharge	0—No functional mobility	<0.001	29.9 (24.1–35.7)	<0.001
	1—Dependent in mobility level 2		18.0 (11.8–24.2)	<0.001
	2—Dependent in mobility level 1		12.0 (7.1–17.0)	<0.001
	3—Independent mobility under supervision		3.6 (−1.2–8.5)	0.141
	4—Independent mobility on a flat surface		ref.	
FMS at hospital discharge	1—Freely mobile without aids 2—Mobile outdoors with one aid 3—Mobile outdoors with two aids or frame 4—Some indoor mobility but never goes outside without help 5—No functional mobility	0.014		
Katz-ADL6 at hospital discharge		<0.001		
Rehabilitation department skilled nursing home	Skilled nursing home A Skilled nursing home B Skilled nursing home C	<0.001		

* Univariate analysis was performed using a Spearman correlation analysis for continuous variables and a Mann–Whitney U or Kruskal–Wallis test for categorical variables. *p*, *p*-value; ref., reference; (P)FMS, (Pre-)Fracture Mobility Score; Katz-ADL, Katz Index of Independence in Activities of Daily Living; CCI, Charlson Comorbidity Index; ASA, American Society of Anesthesiologists physical status classification; SNAQ, Short Nutritional Assessment Questionnaire; Hb, hemoglobin; PFNA, Proximal Femoral Nail Antirotation; DHS, Dynamic Hip Screw; FAC, Functional Ambulation Categories.

Although the length of geriatric rehabilitation stay was not normally distributed, the residual plot of the multivariate linear regression model did show a normal distribution. Therefore, the multivariate linear regression analysis was still the appropriate analysis to use. Age, premorbid living situation, the need for climbing stairs, PFMS, premorbid Katz-ADL6, ASA score, surgical treatment, postoperative weight-bearing protocol, in-hospital anemia, in-hospital heart failure, in-hospital delirium, uncomplicated hospital course, FAC at hospital discharge, and Katz-ADL6 at hospital discharge were included in the multivariate linear regression model. Because hip fracture type was strongly associated with surgical treatment, it was not included in the model. Surgical treatment was regarded to be more patient-specific, as it depends on both the type of fracture and the condition of the patient. FMS at hospital discharge was also not included in the model as it was strongly associated with FACs at hospital discharge. The FAC was considered more relevant in the transmural care pathway compared to the FMS because it is more widely used in geriatric rehabilitation departments to assess patient progress. Furthermore, the rehabilitation department of the skilled nursing homes was not included in the model due to its association with the FAC at hospital discharge. Skilled nursing home A had the highest percentage of patients with a lower FAC at hospital discharge compared to skilled nursing homes B and C within their respective populations. This was a coincidence, as the skilled nursing home placement procedure does not depend on the FAC. The FAC was considered more relevant compared to the rehabilitation department of skilled nursing homes because the FAC is clinically more relevant.

The final multivariate model included the following variables: FAC at hospital discharge, premorbid living situation, postoperative weight-bearing protocol, surgical treatment, in-hospital delirium, and in-hospital heart failure (Table 2). FAC 0 (B = 29.9, 95% CI 24.1–35.7), FAC 1 (B = 18.0, 95% CI 11.8–24.2), FAC 2 (B = 12.0, 95% CI 7.1–17.0), or FAC 3 (B = 3.6, 95% CI −1.2–9.4) at hospital discharge versus (vs.) FAC 4, living independently with home care services (B = 5.9, 95% CI 2.5–9.3) or in a residential home prior to the hip fracture (B = 0.2, 95% CI −7.4–7.8) vs. living independently without home care services, non- or partial weight-bearing mobilization vs. full weight-bearing mobilization (B = 15.4, 95% CI 8.5–22.2), internal fixation vs. hemiarthroplasty (B = 4.7, 95% CI 1.4–7.9), in-hospital delirium (B = 7.0, 95% CI 2.2–11.7), and in-hospital heart failure (B = 7.9, 95% CI 0.5–15.3) were independent predictors of a longer geriatric rehabilitation stay. The explained variance of this model was 32.0%.

4. Discussion

Independent predictors for a longer length of geriatric rehabilitation stay were a lower FAC at hospital discharge compared to FAC 4; living independently with home care services prior to the hip fracture compared to living independently without home care services; non- or partial weight-bearing mobilization compared to full weight-bearing mobilization; internal fixation compared to hemiarthroplasty; in-hospital delirium; and in-hospital heart failure.

A substantial amount of research exists on the factors influencing the length of stay after hip fracture surgery. However, many studies focus on factors influencing the length of hospital stay [12–15] or the length of stay in other rehabilitation settings (e.g., private care rehabilitation, in-hospital rehabilitation, or both the acute hospital and rehabilitation phases) [3,12–18], making them difficult to compare with this study. Previously identified predictors for a longer length of geriatric rehabilitation stay include higher age [3,16,18]; trochanteric and subtrochanteric fractures versus intracapsular fractures [3]; complications (wound infection, delirium, urinary tract infection, and pneumonia) [3,16]; comorbidities (Parkinson's disease, diabetes, and dementia) [3,16,18]; independent gait at hospital discharge versus dependent gait [4]; living alone prior to the hip fracture versus living together [5,18]; using mobility aids prior to the hip fracture versus being mobile without aids [5,17]; a lower Barthel score at geriatric rehabilitation admission [5]; a lower Functional Independence Measure score at rehabilitation admission [16]; a lower Abbreviated Mental Test Score [17]; and a higher pain score at rehabilitation admission [18]. Among all these previously identified predictors, this study confirmed that in-hospital delirium is a predictor for a longer length of geriatric rehabilitation stay. Additionally, the previously identified predictor of trochanteric and subtrochanteric fractures versus intracapsular fractures can be compared to the predictor found in this study: internal fixation versus hemiarthroplasty. This is because the type of hip fracture is strongly associated with the choice of surgical treatment. However, this study did not include hip fracture type in the multivariate model, as surgical treatment was considered to be more patient-specific. Furthermore, the previously identified predictor of independent gait at hospital discharge versus dependent gait can be compared to a predictor found in this study: lower FAC at hospital discharge compared to FAC 4. This is because the FAC score also assesses the degree of walking independence of the patient. The remaining previously identified predictors for a longer length of geriatric rehabilitation stay do not align with the predictors found in this study. A possible explanation for this difference is that other studies used small study populations or different rehabilitation settings. The present study utilized a study population of 561 patients, specifically focusing on the length of stay in geriatric rehabilitation departments at skilled nursing homes. Consequently, this study solely examined in-hospital variables and did not include variables from the rehabilitation phase. This decision was made to prioritize the identification of predictors for the length of geriatric rehabilitation stay upon hospital discharge. Using variables from the rehabilitation phase does not allow for the early prediction of the length of geriatric rehabilitation stay. This hinders healthcare professionals from creating appropriate therapy schedules and preparing patients for what to expect during the rehabilitation period. Another explanation may be that this study assessed the comorbidity burden using the CCI, rather than assessing the specific types of comorbidities as possible predictors. This means that from this study, it is not clear if specific comorbidities may be predictors for the length of geriatric rehabilitation stay. However, this study chose to use the CCI because it captures not only the presence of comorbidities but also their severity, which may be more comprehensive than considering individual comorbidities alone [9].

Each identified independent predictor contributes to a longer length of geriatric rehabilitation stay in specific ways. For patients with a lower FAC at hospital discharge, functional self-reliance may be achieved more slowly, resulting in a longer length of geriatric rehabilitation stay. This highlights the importance of early mobilization during the hospital phase, as it enhances the functional recovery of patients [19–21]. Patients who lived independently with home care services prior to the hip fracture may require more complex care due to their decreased resilience. Although home care services offer some level of support, they may not fully address their rehabilitation needs following hip fracture surgery. As a result, these patients may require a longer length of geriatric rehabilitation stay. Receiving home care services following geriatric rehabilitation for patients who lived independently without home care services prior to the hip fracture may provide sufficient support and assistance to shorten the length of geriatric rehabilitation stay. Patients who lived in a residential home prior to the hip fracture may have sufficient support and assistance available at the residential home to shorten the length of geriatric rehabilitation stay. Patients with non- or partial weight-bearing mobilization are unable to mobilize or have a limited ability to do so and because of this situation receive a lower frequency of therapy during the first six weeks of rehabilitation. This results in a longer length of geriatric rehabilitation stay because their progress in regaining mobility and independence is slower. This is consistent with previous studies that have identified a relationship between a reduced length of hospital stay following hip fracture surgery and full weight-bearing mobilization [22,23]. Patients who undergo internal fixation may experience more post-operative pain and may require longer periods of non- or partial weight-bearing mobilization compared to those who undergo hemiarthroplasty [24,25]. This is due to the nature of the procedures: Hemiarthroplasty involves replacing the fractured hip with a prosthetic implant, whereas internal fixation involves stabilizing the fractured hip using intramedullary nails, plates, and/or screws. In-hospital delirium is characterized by symptoms such as cognitive impairment. Patients who develop an in-hospital delirium are less likely to mobilize after hip fracture surgery [26], which requires more time-intensive medical and nursing care. Similarly, patients with in-hospital heart failure face limitations during rehabilitation due to symptoms such as fatigue, reduced exercise capacity, dyspnea, and hypotension [14], also necessitating more time-intensive medical and nursing care. These findings are consistent with previous studies that have identified relationships between an extended length of hospital stay following hip fractures and either heart failure or delirium [14,27–29].

The results of this study are the first step towards a more efficient rehabilitation pathway. The length of geriatric rehabilitation stay can be better predicted upon hospital discharge, enabling patients to be better prepared for what to expect during the rehabilitation period. Furthermore, this information makes it possible to identify patients who may rehabilitate more quickly. This group may benefit from a more intensive therapy schedule to facilitate even faster recovery. Since early mobilization during the hospital phase enhances the functional recovery of patients, increasing the intensity of therapy early in postoperative rehabilitation may also contribute to faster recovery among other groups [19–21]. Shorter geriatric rehabilitation stays can address potential future capacity issues, as a faster patient flow will enable the treatment of an increasing number of patients with hip fractures.

The limitation of our study is the lack of information on cognitive functioning prior to admission to the geriatric rehabilitation department. No tests measuring cognitive functioning were conducted during the hospital phase. The presence of an in-hospital delirium is the only cognitive functioning status we assessed. However, cognitive functioning may significantly influence the length of geriatric rehabilitation stay, as patients with cognitive impairments may have difficulty performing physiotherapy exercises. A strength of our study lies in the inclusion of a great diversity of possible predictors from both the physical and social domains in the analyses of predictors for the length of geriatric rehabilitation stay. Furthermore, our results statistically confirm the independent predictors for a prolonged length of geriatric rehabilitation stay at skilled nursing homes. These predictors were previously thought to influence the length of stay based on clinical experience but lacked statistical proof. In addition, this study distinguishes itself by focusing exclusively on in-hospital variables, allowing for the early prediction of the length of geriatric rehabilitation stay. Lastly, this study is also valuable for developing a final prediction model in which the length of geriatric rehabilitation stay can be predicted at the time of hospital discharge; something that cannot be achieved with clinical experience alone.

The explained variance of 32.0% in the multivariate model showed that other predictors for length of rehabilitation stay exist that were not included in the present study. Therefore, future research is recommended to optimize the multivariate model. Additional factors that are considered important in predicting the length of geriatric rehabilitation stay should be incorporated. Since early mobilization and physical activity enhance the functional recovery of patients [19–21], continuously monitored physical activity using a sensor during the in-hospital phase is relevant to add to the model. Other relevant factors to add to the model are cognitive functioning assessed with a cognitive screening test during the hospital phase and the fear of falling. Fear of falling could influence the length of geriatric rehabilitation stay, as it may impede rehabilitation by being associated with anxiety and self-efficacy [30]. The occurrence of complications during the rehabilitation stay could also influence the length of the rehabilitation stay [3]. However, this factor cannot be included in the analysis to predict the length of rehabilitation stay upon hospital discharge.

5. Conclusions

A lower FAC at hospital discharge vs. FAC 4, living independently with home care services prior to the hip fracture vs. living independently without home care services, non- or partial weight-bearing mobilization vs. full weight-bearing mobilization, internal fixation vs. hemiarthroplasty, in-hospital delirium, and in-hospital heart failure were found as independent predictors of a longer length of geriatric rehabilitation stay. These results are the first step towards a more efficient rehabilitation pathway. However, with an explained variance of 32.0% in the multivariate model, there are more predictors of a longer length of stay that were not included in this study. Future investigations will be needed to identify additional predictors to better predict the length of geriatric rehabilitation stay upon hospital discharge. The ability to predict the length of geriatric rehabilitation stay more precisely will help healthcare professionals prepare patients for what to expect during the rehabilitation period and create appropriate therapy schedules, aiming for faster recovery. This may address potential future capacity issues, as a faster patient flow will enable the treatment of an increasing number of patients with hip fractures.

Author Contributions: Conceptualization, S.M.K., S.W., D.v.D., M.V., M.M.R.V.-H. and J.H.H.; methodology, S.M.K., S.W., D.v.D. and M.V.; software, S.M.K. and S.W.; formal analysis, S.M.K.; investigation, S.M.K. and S.W.; resources, S.M.K. and S.W.; data curation, S.M.K., S.W., D.v.D. and Up&Go after a Hip Fracture Group; writing—original draft preparation, S.M.K. and S.W.; writing—review and editing, S.M.K., S.W., D.v.D., M.V., M.M.R.V.-H. and J.H.H.; visualization, S.M.K.; supervision, D.v.D. and J.H.H.; project administration, S.M.K. All authors have read and agreed to the published version of the manuscript.

Funding: This research received no external funding.

Institutional Review Board Statement: The study was conducted in accordance with the Declaration of Helsinki and approved by the Institutional Review Board of Ziekenhuisgroep Twente, Almelo, the Netherlands (ZGT17-40, date of latest approval 20 February 2024).

Informed Consent Statement: Informed consent was obtained from all subjects involved in the study.

Data Availability Statement: Data are unavailable due to privacy restrictions.

Acknowledgments: The authors would like to thank the healthcare professionals of the rehabilitation departments of the nursing home institutions Carintreggeland, TriviumMeulenbeltZorg, and ZorgAccent for their contribution to the transmural Up&Go after the hip fracture project.

Conflicts of Interest: The authors declare no conflicts of interest.

References

1. van Dartel, D.; Vermeer, M.; Folbert, E.C.; Arends, A.J.; Vollenbroek-Hutten, M.M.R.; Hegeman, J.H. Early Predictors for Discharge to Geriatric Rehabilitation after Hip Fracture Treatment of Older Patients. *J. Am. Med. Dir. Assoc.* **2021**, *22*, 2454–2460. [CrossRef] [PubMed]
2. Nijmeijer, W.S.; van Dartel, D.; de Groot, R.; Woudsma, S.; Folbert, E.C.; den Braber, N.; Vermeer, M.; Hegeman, J.H.; Vollenbroek-Hutten, M.M. Transparency in hip fracture recovery over institutional boundaries: The transmural monitoring pathway. *Clin. Rehabil.* **2023**, *37*, 1406–1419. [CrossRef] [PubMed]
3. Ireland, A.W.; Kelly, P.J.; Cumming, R.G. Total hospital stay for hip fracture: Measuring the variations due to pre-fracture residence, rehabilitation, complications and comorbidities. *BMC Health Serv. Res.* **2015**, *15*, 17. [CrossRef] [PubMed]
4. Adrados, M.; Wang, K.; Deng, Y.; Bozzo, J.; Messina, T.; Stevens, A.; Moore, A.; Morris, J.; O'Connor, M.I. A Simple Physical Therapy Algorithm Is Successful in Decreasing Skilled Nursing Facility Length of Stay and Increasing Cost Savings after Hip Fracture with No Increase in Adverse Events. *Geriatr. Orthop. Surg. Rehabil.* **2021**, *12*, 2151459321998615. [CrossRef]
5. Fault, L.; van Schieveen, C.; Schalk, B.W.M. Met een heupfractuur op de Geriatrische Revalidatie: Factoren gerelateerd aan een kortere opnameduur. *Tijdschr. Ouderengeneeskunde* **2021**, *5*, 16–27.
6. International Organization for Standardization. Information Security, Cybersecurity and Privacy Protection-Information Security Management Systems-Requirements (ISO/IEC Standard No. 27001). 2022. Available online: https://www.iso.org/standard/27001#amendment (accessed on 15 June 2024).
7. Holden, M.K.; Gill, K.M.; Magliozzi, M.R.; Nathan, J.; Piehl-Baker, L. Clinical gait assessment in the neurologically impaired. Reliability and meaningfulness. *Phys. Ther.* **1984**, *64*, 35–40. [CrossRef]
8. Katz, S.; Ford, A.B.; Moskowitz, R.W.; Jackson, B.A.; Jaffe, M.W. Studies of illness in the aged. The index of ADL: A standardized measure of biological and psychosocial function. *JAMA* **1963**, *185*, 914–919. [CrossRef]
9. Charlson, M.E.; Pompei, P.; Ales, K.L.; MacKenzie, C.R. A new method of classifying prognostic comorbidity in longitudinal studies: Development and validation. *J. Chronic Dis.* **1987**, *40*, 373–383. [CrossRef]
10. Keats, A.S. The ASA classification of physical status—A recapitulation. *Anesthesiology* **1978**, *49*, 233–236. [CrossRef]
11. Kruizenga, H.M.; Seidell, J.C.; de Vet, H.C.; Wierdsma, N.J.; van Bokhorst-de van der Schueren, M.A. Development and validation of a hospital screening tool for malnutrition: The short nutritional assessment questionnaire (SNAQ). *Clin. Nutr.* **2005**, *24*, 75–82. [CrossRef]
12. Unnanuntana, A.; Anusitviwat, C.; Lertsiripatarajit, V.; Riawraengsattha, P.; Raksakietisak, M. Early Hip Fracture Surgery within 24 h did not Reduce the Mortality Rate but Resulted in Less Postoperative Opioid use and a Shorter Length of Stay: A Retrospective Study of 276 Patients from a Tertiary Private Hospital in Thailand. *Geriatr. Orthop. Surg. Rehabil.* **2024**, *15*, 21514593241250150. [CrossRef] [PubMed]
13. Raksakietisak, M.; Lurngnateetape, A.; Riansuwan, K.; Noiwan, N.; Chaiyarak, C.; Keawmoon, K.; von Bormann, B. Patients with osteoporotic hip fractures: Factors affecting length of hospital stay (LOS) and outcome. *J. Med. Assoc. Thai* **2012**, *95*, 917–924. [PubMed]
14. Liu, H.; Xing, F.; Jiang, J.; Chen, Z.; Xiang, Z.; Duan, X. Random forest predictive modeling of prolonged hospital length of stay in elderly hip fracture patients. *Front. Med.* **2024**, *11*, 1362153. [CrossRef] [PubMed]
15. Siminiuc, D.; Gumuskaya, O.; Mitchell, R.; Bell, J.; Cameron, I.D.; Hallen, J.; Birkenhead, K.; Hurring, S.; Baxter, B.; Close, J.; et al. Rehabilitation after surgery for hip fracture—The impact of prompt, frequent and mobilisation-focused physiotherapy on discharge outcomes: An observational cohort study. *BMC Geriatr.* **2024**, *24*, 629. [CrossRef]
16. Thornburgh, Z.; Samuel, D. Factors Influencing Length of Stay and Discharge Destination of Patients with Hip Fracture Rehabilitating in a Private Care Setting. *Geriatrics* **2022**, *7*, 44. [CrossRef] [PubMed]
17. Richards, T.; Glendenning, A.; Benson, D.; Alexander, S.; Thati, S. The independent patient factors that affect length of stay following hip fractures. *Ann. R. Coll. Surg. Engl.* **2018**, *100*, 556–562. [CrossRef] [PubMed]
18. Daly, N.; Fortin, C.; Jaglal, S.; MacDonald, S.L. Predictors of Exceeding Target Inpatient Rehabilitation Length of Stay After Hip Fracture. *Am. J. Phys. Med. Rehabil.* **2020**, *99*, 630–635. [CrossRef]
19. Riemen, A.H.; Hutchison, J.D. The multidisciplinary management of hip fractures in older patients. *Orthop. Trauma* **2016**, *30*, 117–122. [CrossRef]

20. Morri, M.; Forni, C.; Marchioni, M.; Bonetti, E.; Marseglia, F.; Cotti, A. Which factors are independent predictors of early recovery of mobility in the older adults' population after hip fracture? A cohort prognostic study. *Arch. Orthop. Trauma Surg.* **2018**, *138*, 35–41. [CrossRef]
21. van Dartel, D.; Wang, Y.; Hegeman, J.H.; Vermeer, M.; Vollenbroek-Hutten, M.M.R. Patterns of physical activity over time in older patients rehabilitating after hip fracture surgery: A preliminary observational study. *BMC Geriatr.* **2023**, *23*, 373. [CrossRef]
22. Cunningham, B.P.; Ali, A.; Parikh, H.R.; Heare, A.; Blaschke, B.; Zaman, S.; Montalvo, R.; Reahl, B.; Rotuno, G.; Kark, J.; et al. Immediate weight bearing as tolerated (WBAT) correlates with a decreased length of stay post intramedullary fixation for subtrochanteric fractures: A multicenter retrospective cohort study. *Eur. J. Orthop. Surg. Traumatol.* **2021**, *31*, 235–243. [CrossRef] [PubMed]
23. Kuru, T.; Olçar, H.A. Effects of early mobilization and weight bearing on postoperative walking ability and pain in geriatric patients operated due to hip fracture: A retrospective analysis. *Turk. J. Med. Sci.* **2020**, *50*, 117–125. [PubMed]
24. Gjertsen, J.E.; Vinje, T.; Lie, S.A.; Engesaeter, L.B.; Havelin, L.I.; Furnes, O.; Fevang, J.M. Patient satisfaction, pain, and quality of life 4 months after displaced femoral neck fractures: A comparison of 663 fractures treated with internal fixation and 906 with bipolar hemiarthroplasty reported to the Norwegian Hip Fracture Register. *Acta Orthop.* **2008**, *79*, 594–601. [CrossRef] [PubMed]
25. Salpakoski, A.; Kallinen, M.; Kiviranta, I.; Alen, M.; Portegijs, E.; Jämsen, E.; Ylinen, J.; Rantanen, T.; Sipilä, S. Type of surgery is associated with pain and walking difficulties among older people with previous hip fracture. *Geriatr. Gerontol. Int.* **2016**, *16*, 754–761. [CrossRef]
26. Said, C.M.; Delahunt, M.; Ciavarella, V.; Al Maliki, D.; Boys, A.M.; Vogrin, S.; Berney, S. Factors Impacting Early Mobilization Following Hip Fracture: An Observational Study. *J. Geriatr. Phys. Ther.* **2021**, *44*, 88–93. [CrossRef]
27. Cullen, M.W.; Gullerud, R.E.; Larson, D.R.; Melton, L.J., 3rd; Huddleston, J.M. Impact of heart failure on hip fracture outcomes: A population-based study. *J. Hosp. Med.* **2011**, *6*, 507–512. [CrossRef]
28. Lee, S.J.; Jung, S.H.; Lee, S.U.; Lim, J.Y.; Yoon, K.S.; Lee, S.Y. Postoperative delirium after hip surgery is a potential risk factor for incident dementia: A systematic review and meta-analysis of prospective studies. *Arch. Gerontol. Geriatr.* **2020**, *87*, 103977. [CrossRef]
29. Zhao, S.; Sun, T.; Zhang, J.; Chen, X.; Wang, X. Risk factors and prognosis of postoperative delirium in nonagenarians with hip fracture. *Sci. Rep.* **2023**, *13*, 2167. [CrossRef] [PubMed]
30. Visschedijk, J.; van Balen, R.; Hertogh, C.; Achterberg, W. Fear of falling in patients with hip fractures: Prevalence and related psychological factors. *J. Am. Med. Dir. Assoc.* **2013**, *14*, 218–220. [CrossRef]

Journal of
Clinical Medicine

MDPI

Article

Variability in Care Pathways for Hip Fracture Patients in The Netherlands

Hanne-Eva van Bremen [1,2,3,4], Thamar Kroes [5], Lotta J. Seppala [3,4], Emma A. Gans [6,7], Johannes H. Hegeman [8,9], Nathalie van der Velde [3,4] and Hanna C. Willems [1,3,4,*]

1 Amsterdam Bone Center, Movement Sciences Amsterdam, Meibergdreef 9, 1105 AZ Amsterdam, The Netherlands; h.vanbremen@amsterdamumc.nl
2 Dutch Institute for Clinical Auditing, Rijnsburgerweg 10, 2333 AA Leiden, The Netherlands
3 Section of Geriatric Medicine, Department of Internal Medicine, Amsterdam UMC, Meibergdreef 9, 1105 AZ Amsterdam, The Netherlands; l.j.seppala@amsterdamumc.nl (L.J.S.); n.vandervelde@amsterdamumc.nl (N.v.d.V.)
4 Amsterdam Public Health Research Institute, Meibergdreef 9, 1105 AZ Amsterdam, The Netherlands
5 Department of Trauma Surgery, St. Antonius Hospital Utrecht–Nieuwegein, 3543 AZ Utrecht, The Netherlands; t.kroes@antoniusziekenhuis.nl
6 University Center of Geriatric Medicine, University Medical Center Groningen, Hanzeplein 1, 9713 GZ Groningen, The Netherlands; e.gans@kennisinstituut.nl
7 Knowledge Institute of the Dutch Association of Medical Specialists, Mercatorlaan 1200, 3528 BL Utrecht, The Netherlands
8 Biomedical Signals and Systems Group, University of Twente, Drienerlolaan 5, 7522 NB Enschede, The Netherlands; h.hegeman@zgt.nl
9 Department of Trauma Surgery, Ziekenhuisgroep Twente, Zilvermeeuw 1, 7909 PP Almelo, The Netherlands
* Correspondence: h.c.willems@amsterdamumc.nl

Abstract: Background/Objectives: Integrated orthogeriatric care has demonstrated benefits in hip fracture management for older patients. Comprehensive care pathways are essential for effective integrated care delivery, yet local variability in care pathways persists. We assessed the current hip fracture care pathways in the Netherlands, focusing on the variability between these care pathways and the degree of implementation of orthogeriatric care. **Methods**: A nationwide inventory study was conducted. A survey was sent to all hospitals in the Netherlands to collect the care pathways or local protocols for hip fracture care. All care elements reported in the care pathways and protocols were systematically analyzed by two independent researchers. Furthermore, an assessment was performed to determine which model of orthogeriatric care was applied. **Results**: All 71 Dutch hospitals were contacted, and 56 hospitals responded (79%), of which 46 (82%) provided a care pathway or protocol. Forty-one care elements were identified in total. In the care pathways and protocols, the variability in the description of these individual care elements ranged from 7% to 87%. Twenty-one hospitals had an integrated care model with shared responsibility, while an equal number followed an orthopedic trauma surgeon-led care model. **Conclusions**: These findings provide a detailed description of the hip fracture care pathways in the Netherlands. Variations were observed concerning the care elements described in the care pathways, the structure of the care pathway, and the specification of several elements. The implementation of integrated care with shared responsibilities, as recommended by the international literature, has not been achieved nationwide. The clinical implications of the variability between care pathways, such as the influence on the quality of care, need to be further investigated.

Keywords: hip fracture; care pathway; integrated hip fracture care

1. Introduction

Integrated orthogeriatric care has significant benefits for older patients with a hip fracture, including improved quality of life, reduced morbidity and mortality, increased activities of daily living at 6 and 12 months, and reduced direct costs in comparison to usual care [1,2]. Hip fracture patients are distinct due to the high prevalence of multimorbidity and increased frailty [3]. These patient characteristics are associated with prolonged hospital stays, delays in surgery, a functional decline, and increased mortality rates [4]. Given these patient characteristics and risk factors, the treatment of hip fracture patients is complex and requires the integration of both surgical and geriatric care to adequately address comorbidities and geriatric syndromes [1].

In the literature, different models of integration in orthogeriatric trauma care are described: (1) orthopedic trauma surgeon-led care with a geriatrician as a consulting physician; (2) geriatrician-led care with consultation from an orthopedic trauma surgeon, and (3) integrated care models with shared responsibilities between a geriatrician and orthopedic trauma surgeon [5–7]. In the integrated care model, orthogeriatric care can be implemented as an integral component of the orthogeriatric ward. This has demonstrated positive effects on both patient outcomes and the quality of care, including reduced lengths of stay in the hospital and emergency department and shorter times to operation [8–10].

The integration of surgical and geriatric care for hip fracture patients is preferably coordinated in care pathways that address both clinical and organizational issues. In the current literature, several synonyms exist for the term 'care pathway', such as clinical pathway, model of care, and integrated care pathway. It is defined as an integrated care plan that outlines patient goals and provides the sequence and timing of the necessary actions to achieve these goals [11,12]. Several care pathways are known for a various number of conditions. The use of care pathways enhances the efficiency and quality of care for hip fracture patients. It can also be used as a method to implement evidence-based clinical guidelines in practice [13].

Despite the added value of care integration in orthogeriatric hip fracture care, the implementation of orthogeriatric care remains inconsistent across hospitals in the Netherlands and between countries in Europe [14,15]. Although a certain level of local variability in care processes across hospitals is inevitable, comprehensive protocols are important for integrated care delivery [16–18]. Therefore, the aim of this study was to assess the current hip fracture care pathways and protocols in the Netherlands for variability between the pathways by evaluating the different elements and the degree of implementation of orthogeriatric care.

2. Materials and Methods

A cross-sectional national inventory study was conducted from 1 May 2023 until 1 October 2023. All hospitals across the Netherlands were asked to provide their protocols regarding hip fracture care. If the hospitals did not respond to the initial request sent through professional organizations, they were contacted directly via telephone and email for their care pathway protocol or protocols for hip fracture patients. Recognizing the multidisciplinary care approach, both the geriatric and surgical departments were asked to provide the documents. All protocols that specifically addressed the treatment of hip fracture patients were included. Additional information per email and personal experiences shared by healthcare professionals were excluded from the analysis as the scope of this study focused on the assessment of local authorized protocols and care pathways.

2.1. Data Analysis

2.1.1. Screening Tool

No validated method was available for the evaluation of local care pathways. Previous research into systematic reviews assessing the quality of care pathways did not establish a gold standard for screening [19]. When asked for a recommendation by researchers in the field, the European Pathway Association (EPA) stated that there are currently no suitable tools for the comparison of local (hip fracture) protocols or care pathways.

In the absence of a validated method, a manifest content analysis was conducted on all retrieved protocols [20]. This entailed (1) the identification of the care elements within the care pathways and (2) examining what was documented about the care elements across the care pathways. Within several care elements, variability was observed and further explored, encompassing the type of diagnostics (emergency care), treatment team, use of thrombosis prophylaxis, involvement of paramedics (pre- and post-operative), and organization of outpatient visits.

2.1.2. Content Analysis

The content analysis was conducted using alternate deductive and inductive methods. Efforts were made to ensure the robustness of the approach. Before the analysis, a content model of care elements was established based on the national Dutch hip fracture care guidelines [21]. This content model was modified and approved by an expert panel including geriatricians, internists, orthopedic surgeons, trauma surgeons, and physiotherapists. After the content model was established, two researchers (H.B. and T.K.) independently screened all protocols and noted the presence of care elements in a deductive manner. Furthermore, the researchers used this initial screening to reveal the content of the care elements and identify additional care elements in an inductive manner. After intercoder agreement was achieved (H.B., T.K., H.W.), several care elements were added to the content model. A second screening was conducted to note both the inclusion and content of the newly identified care elements in all protocols (H.B., T.K.). After the second round, the independent evaluations were assessed for differences, and inter-coder agreement was reached (H.B., T.K.). In instances of non-agreement, a third researcher (H.W.) was available to resolve discrepancies.

The intention was to categorize the care elements according to Donabedian's healthcare quality model to identify the protocols' structural, process, and outcome elements [22]. However, all identified care elements were process-related. Consequently, the researchers chose to report the care elements by following the care pathway of the Orthogeriatric Care Model of the FFN, encompassing the emergency phase, pre-operative phase, operative phase, post-operative phase, rehabilitation, and return to function [23]. A non-operative phase was added separately since it recurred in several care pathways. Structural elements were identified within the care pathways: in- and exclusion criteria, the use of quality indicators, and responsibility tables or flowcharts.

2.1.3. Model of Orthogeriatric Care

The type of integrated care in orthogeriatric trauma was divided into three different types: (1) orthopedic trauma surgeon-led care—a surgeon-led model with the patient on an orthopedic/surgical ward and consultation with the geriatrician; (2) geriatrician-led care—a geriatrician-led model with the patient on a geriatric ward and consultation with an orthopedic trauma surgeon; (3) an integrated care model with shared responsibility—the patient on a ward with shared care between a geriatrician and orthopedic trauma surgeon [5–7]. The model used in the hospital/care pathway was identified and independently described by the two researchers (H.B., T.K.). In case of disagreement, a third researcher (H.W.) was available.

3. Results

3.1. Inventory

Out of 71 contacted hospitals, 56 responded (response rate 79%). Among them, 46 (82%) hospitals shared their care pathways. Four of the responding hospitals were affiliated with universities. Ten hospitals could not provide a care pathway: two had a care pathway under development, three did not have one, four hospitals did not share a written protocol but instead provided information via telephone and details about the organization, and one declined to provide it. For 44 hospitals, the type of orthogeriatric care model could be identified. The distribution was equal between hospitals with orthopedic trauma surgeon-led care (N = 21) and those with an integrated care model with shared responsibilities (N = 21). Two hospitals had geriatrician-led care (Figure 1).

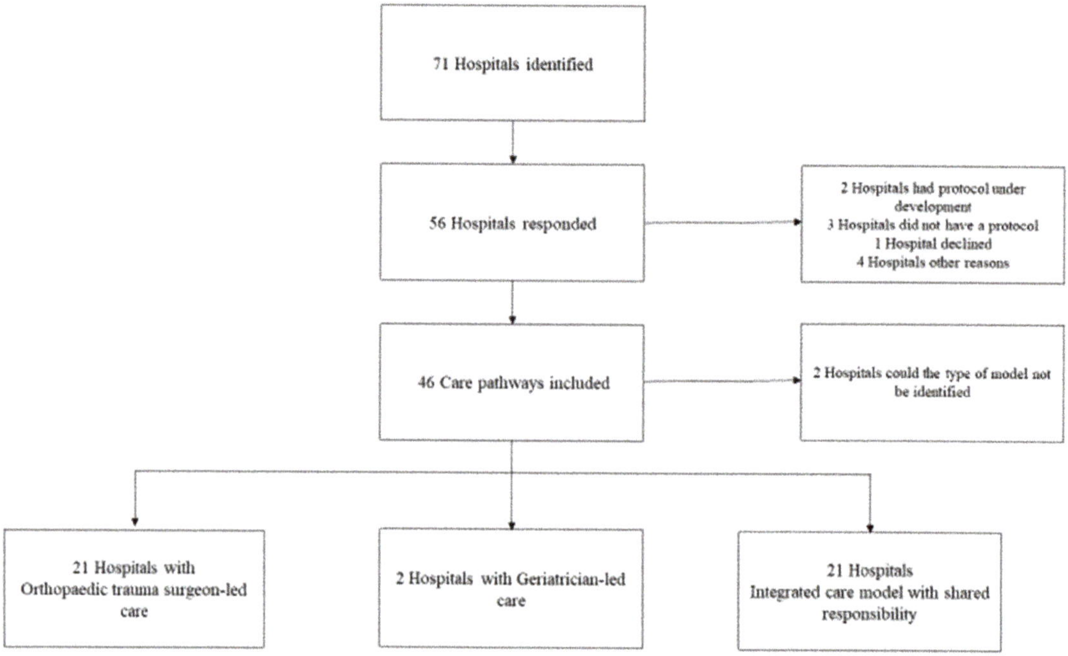

Figure 1. Flowchart with the inventory process and distribution of orthogeriatric care models.

3.2. Identified Care Elements

A detailed overview of the care elements with a description of the content is provided in Figure 2. In total, 43 care elements were identified by the content analysis. The presence of the care elements varied between 7% (information–expectation management in the non-operative phase) and 87% (delirium prevention/risk analysis) (Figure 3). Several elements were present in >70% of the hip fracture care pathways, including pain management, medical assessment—blood tests and electrocardiograms, a urinary catheterization policy, thrombosis prophylaxis, delirium prevention/risk analysis, discharge planning, and a mobilization policy (Table 1). Various care elements were present in less than 20% of the hip fracture care pathways, including pain management in the non-operative phase, the involvement of carers and/or family, and information/expectation management in the non-operative phase.

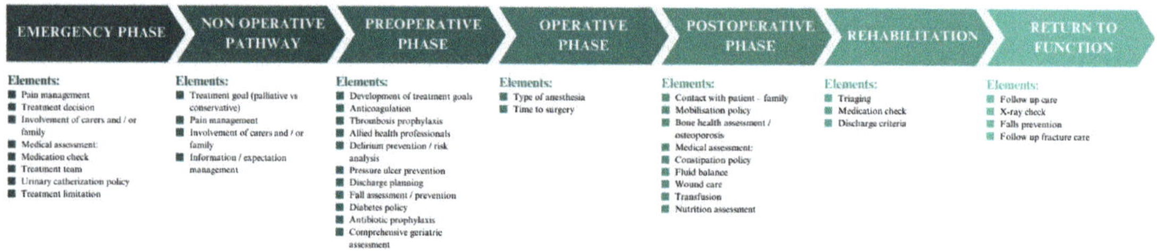

Figure 2. Overview of identified care elements per phase of care.

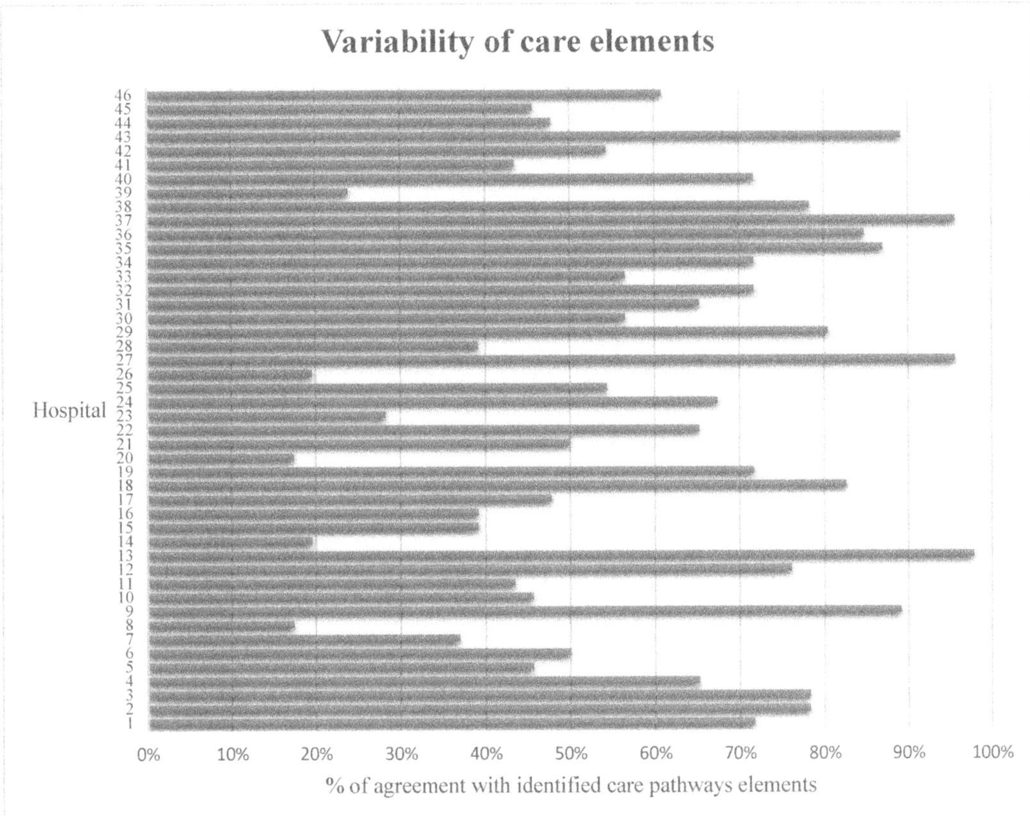

Figure 3. Percentage of agreement with the identified care elements per hospital.

Table 1. Overview of identified care elements.

Phase	Elements of Care Pathways	Total *N* = 46 *N* (%)
Emergency phase	Pain management	35 (76)
	Treatment decision	28 (61)
	Involvement of carers and/or family	18 (39)
	Medical assessment:	
	chest X-ray	27 (59)
	urine analysis	17 (37)
	blood test	38 (83)
	electrocardiogram	35 (76)
	Medication check	24 (52)
	Treatment team	
	attending physician	17 (37)
	consulting physician	12 (26)
	Urinary catherization policy	33 (72)
	Treatment limitation	29 (63)

Table 1. *Cont.*

Phase	Elements of Care Pathways	Total *N* = 46 *N* (%)
Non-operative pathway	Treatment goal (palliative vs. conservative)	17 (37)
	Pain management	7 (15)
	Involvement of carers and/or family	5 (11)
	Information/expectation management	3 (7)
Pre-operative phase	Development of treatment goals	20 (43)
	Anticoagulation	25 (54)
	Thrombosis prophylaxis	36 (78)
	Allied health professionals physiotherapist dietician	 29 (63) 20 (43)
	Delirium prevention/risk analysis	40 (87)
	Pressure ulcer prevention	27 (59)
	Discharge planning	37 (80)
	Fall assessment/prevention	30 (65)
	Diabetes policy	12 (26)
	Antibiotic prophylaxis	19 (41)
	Comprehensive geriatric assessment	10 (22)
Operative phase	Type of anesthesia	10 (22)
	Time to surgery	18 (39)
Post-operative phase	Contact with patient/family	25 (54)
	Mobilization policy	33 (72)
	Bone health assessment/osteoporosis	25 (54)
	Medical assessment: X-ray blood test	 22 (48) 19 (41)
	Constipation policy	18 (39)
	Fluid balance	26 (57)
	Wound care	26 (57)
	Transfusion	16 (35)
	Nutrition assessment	27 (59)
Rehabilitation	Triaging	31 (67)
	Medication check	22 (48)
	Discharge criteria	10 (22)
Return to function	Follow-up care two weeks six weeks three months	 13 (28) 26 (57) 19 (41)
	X-ray check	21 (46)
	Fall prevention	16 (35)
	Follow-up fracture care	28 (61)

3.3. Structure of Care Pathway

The care pathways varied in their inclusion and exclusion criteria and the use of quality indicators. Several care pathways applied an age threshold for patients ≥ 70 years old (N = 7) or only included frail patients (N = 4), and four care pathways excluded pathological hip fractures.

Out of 46 care pathways, 19 described quality indicators. An overview of the identified quality indicators can be found in Table 2. The quality indicator "Operation within 24 h after admission" was most often described (N = 9). Flowcharts and responsibility formats were identified as structural elements. Specifically, 11 included a flowchart of the care pathway, and eight included a responsibility matrix specifying which healthcare provider was responsible for each part of the care.

3.4. Care Elements

3.4.1. Diagnostics (Emergency Care)

Among the 46 care pathways, 39 described information regarding the medical assessment conducted in the Emergency Department. Various types of diagnostics were identified, including chest X-rays, electrocardiograms, blood tests, and urine sediment analyses. Specifically, 38 hospitals recommended blood tests, 35 mentioned electrocardiograms, 27 described chest X-rays, and 17 specified urine sediment analyses.

3.4.2. Treatment Team

The attending physician was, in most cases, the orthopedic surgeon or a trauma-certified surgeon (N = 16), and the geriatrician was the consulting physician (N = 15). In limited cases, the geriatrician acted as an attending physician (N = 2). In some care pathways, a change in the treatment team occurred during the hospital stay, where the geriatrician took over the role of the attending physician from the surgeon after 24 h (N = 1), directly post-operatively (N = 2), or after two days (N = 3).

3.4.3. Use of Thrombosis Prophylaxis

Different types and durations of thrombosis prophylaxis post-operatively were observed in 35 care pathways. In most cases, a separate care protocol was described for the use of thrombosis prophylaxis (N = 8). Dalteparin was mentioned most often (N = 8), with durations varying from 5 weeks (N = 4) to 6 weeks (N = 1). Seven care pathways advised the use of Fraxiparine for 4 to 6 weeks, and two recommended Nadroparin.

3.4.4. Involvement of Allied Health Professionals (Pre- and Post-Operative)

Out of the 46 care pathways, 33 described the consultation of paramedics either pre- or post-operatively. Four types of paramedics were identified: physiotherapy, dietetics, speech therapy, and occupational therapy. Regarding physiotherapy, four care pathways recommended a pre-operative consultation, 13 care pathways a post-operative consultation, and 24 did not specify the timing of consultation. A dietetics consultation was recommended, in most cases, in the case of malnutrition (N = 16). Six care pathways described the consultation of a speech therapist, and one care pathway described the consultation of an occupational therapist.

3.4.5. Outpatient Visits

Among the 46 care pathways, the timing of the outpatient visits could be identified in 34 pathways. Most recommended a follow-up visit six weeks post-operatively (N = 24), and 19 care pathways advised a follow-up visit at three months. Other care pathways advised to plan a visit at 8–10 weeks (N = 1), six months (N = 2), and 12 months (N = 2). Three care pathways recommended to forego outpatient follow-up in the hospital in case the patient was discharged to a nursing home. Two care pathways recommended to forego follow-up in case of cognitive impairment or dementia.

Table 2. Identified quality indicators used in the care pathways.

	Quality Indicators	N
Process	Discharge from the emergency department to a ward within a	
	1 h timeframe	2
	90 min timeframe	1
	2 h timeframe	6
	Assessed by a doctor within 2 h	1
	Operation within X hours after admission	
	24 h	9
	Within 24 h in case of ASA 1-2	1
	36 h	1
	Median time between operation–admission	1
	Discharge from hospital	
	Length of stay	1
	Discharge on day 4–5	1
	% Delayed length of stay (>day 4)	1
	90% Within length of stay of 6 days	1
	Co-treatment by a geriatrician	
	Patients operated by a certified trauma surgeon or orthopedic surgeon and peri-operative co-management by a geriatrician	1
	Co-management in patients over 70 years old	1
	100% assessment by a geriatrician within 1 day of admission	1
	Registry	
	Registration of functional outcome measurement three months after discharge	1
	Registration of functional outcome measurements for patients over 70 years old	1
	Registration of functional measurements before admission and three months after discharge	1
	Percentage of patients with an FICB	
Outcome	Reoperation	
	Within three months due to wound infection	1
	Within 60 days in patients over 65 years old	1
	Informed consent check 100%	1
	Complications (wound infection, pressure ulcer, delirium)	1
	Mortality after 30 days and after one year	1
	Pain score NRS 4	1
	Readmissions (not further specified)	1
	Surgery report within 24 h	1
	Discharge letter within 24 h	1
	Morbidity (not further specified)	1
	Patients aged 50–80 and over 80 with a bone mineral density (BMD) measurement within 1 year before or up to 3 months after a fracture	1

4. Discussion

A descriptive content analysis was conducted to map the orthogeriatric care integration and variability within care pathways in the Netherlands. Forty-three care elements were identified in 46 different care pathways, with substantial variability in the care pathway elements, ranging from 7% to 87%. Further analysis uncovered variability regarding the treatment team, the involvement of allied health professionals, thrombosis management, and post-operative care. The models of orthogeriatric care were divided equally between orthopedic trauma surgeon-led care with geriatric consultation ($N = 21$) and integrated care with shared responsibilities ($N = 21$).

Standardizing clinical processes is an effective strategy in reducing variability and minimizing the risk of medical errors [24]. In this study, substantial variability was observed in several aspects of the care pathways. The variation in care elements as well as treatment policies might therefore be concerning. For example, certain elements, such as delirium prevention, urinary catheterization policies, and discharge planning, occurred relatively frequently, while osteoporosis care was seldom described. Hip fracture patients constitute a heterogeneous group where a uniform approach to care may not always be appropriate. However, it can be argued that certain elements warrant almost universal application, such as having integrated or shared decision-making and a pain management plan, as advocated for by the FFN. Several of these elements, where universal application could be argued, were infrequently described in the care pathways, including the development of treatment goals. Although some space for variability in the clinical application of care is necessary due to the heterogeneity of the hip fracture population, the further standardization of hip fracture care pathways might be a promising improvement strategy.

A prerequisite for the further standardization of hip fracture care pathways is a clear definition of the term 'care pathway'. This is necessary to provide direction for clinicians and establish the grounds for the adequate evaluation of care pathways. In the current literature, several synonyms and definitions exist for the term 'care pathway', and clear descriptions of the care pathway evaluation criteria are lacking. The broad terminology used for the term care pathway also complicates the process of identifying the relevant literature and evaluation methods. To our knowledge, a validated method to evaluate care pathways remains absent. Most literature describes single-site implementations and the implementation of care pathways. It does not examine multiple care pathways on a broad scale, as was conducted in the current study, which looked at the national level. A previous systematic review by Vanhaecht identified various tools to assess care pathways [25]. This review identified the Integrated Care Pathways Appraisal Tool (ICPAT) as the most appropriate tool to evaluate clinical pathway documents; however, it was neither available nor used in practice and mainly focused on the English care setting rather than the Dutch [26,27]. Vanhaecht et al. concluded that extremely little research has been conducted on these tools. The available tools often have a specific application for the implementation and evaluation of the care pathway, work in a particular setting, or are not validated or widely used. Since no validated method was available, the deductive and inductive content analysis made it possible to evaluate all available care pathways critically and understand the variability between the care elements. Therefore, all efforts were made to sustain a robust and valid method for the assessment of the care pathways through evaluation by two independent researchers and contacting the European Pathway Association (EPA) for alternatives.

Besides the ambiguous definition of the term care pathway and the subsequent complicated evaluation, there remains a gap in understanding how care pathways and protocols translate into everyday clinical practice. Consequently, it is unknown how differences within care pathways and protocols between hospitals influence the quality of care. However, the implementation of a care pathway for older patients with hip fractures has been shown to improve the quality of care and is advised by the FFN [28]. As previously described, reducing variability through the standardization of clinical processes, of which a care pathway is one, effectively reduces the risk of medical errors [24]. However, it is important to consider the lessons from the earlier literature that discusses the balance between clinicians' freedom and the autonomy to provide appropriate care [29]. In other words, care pathway implementation does not equal 'cookbook medicine' and this balance is important for successful care pathway implementation.

In this study, almost half of the hospitals in the Netherlands used the integrated care model with shared responsibility. Previous studies favored the integrated care model with shared responsibility and geriatrician-led care over orthopedic trauma surgeon-led care in terms of better outcomes [5–7]. Although the evidence for one model over the other is limited, the overall evidence for orthogeriatric or multidisciplinary care over usual care is apparent. Solberg et al. showed better outcomes for integrated care in comparison to orthopedic trauma surgeon-led care regarding the removal of a urinary catheter, mobilization day one post-operatively, and secondary fracture prevention [30]. In a literature review, Kammerlander et al. compared four different models and found favorable outcomes for integrated care regarding in-hospital mortality, the length of stay, and the mean time to surgery [31]. Van Heghe et al., in a systematic review and meta-analysis, compared the three models used in our study and observed better outcomes for all models in terms of the length of stay, in-hospital mortality, 1-year mortality, and delirium [7]. However, they could not conclusively recommend one orthogeriatric care model over another. Schuijt et al. evaluated the outcomes before and after implementing an integrated orthogeriatric trauma unit and showed a reduction in post-operative complications, lower 1-year mortality, less time spent at the ED, and better data registration [9]. A previous study by Werner et al. found the lowest percentage of joint care in the Netherlands at 74%, compared to the data of other European hip fracture registrations [14]. Since the evidence regarding the benefits of integrated care has been known for several years, this raises the question of why integrated care is not applied in most protocols. The analyzed protocols may provide an incomplete picture of the actual clinical practice due to outdated or incomplete care pathways. Although a previous study found support for integrated care among specialists, including geriatricians and orthopedic trauma surgeons, there may be unknown barriers in the Dutch healthcare system that delay the implementation of integrated care, such as financial reasons or a lack of availability of physicians [32].

The strengths and limitations of this study should be considered. We conducted extensive research looking into local written care pathways in the hospitals, seeking to bridge the gap between the care pathway literature and the real-world hospital setting and explore the gap between the care pathway literature and their implementation in hospitals. The method used in this study made it possible to perform an extensive analysis of the care pathways and elucidate the existing variability. The limitations included the lack of a validated care pathway evaluation method, which resulted in the authors performing a descriptive content analysis. Secondly, we merely explored the documented care pathways and did not evaluate clinical practice. While it is likely that variability in protocols results in variability in clinical practice, this cannot be concluded with certainty.

5. Conclusions

These findings show substantial variability in hip fracture care pathways in the Netherlands. Variations were observed concerning the frequency of care elements described in the care pathways, ranging from 7% to 87%. Additionally, the structure and specifications of specific elements, such as thrombosis prophylaxis and outpatient visits, varied widely. As integrated care with shared responsibilities was observed in less than half of the hospitals, it seems to lag behind in relation to the current scientific recommendations. The clinical implications of the variability between care pathways, such as its influence on the quality of care, need to be further investigated. Future research should focus on developing clear care pathway definitions and evaluation methods.

Author Contributions: Conceptualization, H.-E.v.B., T.K., L.J.S., E.A.G., J.H.H., N.v.d.V. and H.C.W.; Methodology, H.-E.v.B., T.K., L.J.S. and H.C.W. Validation, H.-E.v.B., T.K., L.J.S., E.A.G., J.H.H. and N.v.d.V.; Formal Analysis, H.-E.v.B., T.K. and H.C.W.; Resources, H.-E.v.B., T.K. and H.C.W.; Data Curation, H.-E.v.B., T.K., L.J.S. and H.C.W.; Writing—Original Draft Preparation, H.-E.v.B., T.K., L.J.S., J.H.H., N.v.d.V. and H.C.W.; Writing—Review and Editing, H.-E.v.B., T.K., L.J.S., E.A.G., J.H.H., N.v.d.V. and H.C.W.; Visualization, H.-E.v.B. and T.K.; Supervision, L.J.S., E.A.G., J.H.H., N.v.d.V. and H.C.W.; Project Administration, H.-E.v.B., E.A.G. and H.C.W. All authors have read and agreed to the published version of the manuscript.

Funding: This research received no external funding.

Institutional Review Board Statement: Not applicable.

Informed Consent Statement: Not applicable.

Data Availability Statement: The data presented in this study are available on request from the corresponding author and hospital.

Acknowledgments: The authors would like to thank all participating hospitals that shared the care pathways or protocols.

Conflicts of Interest: The authors declare no conflicts of interest.

References

1. Baroni, M.; Serra, R.; Boccardi, V.; Ercolani, S.; Zengarini, E.; Casucci, P.; Valecchi, R.; Rinonapoli, G.; Caraffa, A.; Mecocci, P.; et al. The Orthogeriatric Comanagement Improves Clinical Outcomes of Hip Fracture in Older Adults. *Osteoporos. Int.* **2019**, *30*, 907–916. [CrossRef] [PubMed]
2. Hsu, Y.F.; Chou, F.H.; Wang, H.H.; Chu, Y.C.; Liao, K.L. Effectiveness of Integrated Care for Elderly Patients with Hip Fractures: A Systematic Review and Meta-Analysis. *Geriatr. Nurs.* **2023**, *49*, 65–73. [CrossRef] [PubMed]
3. Baker, P.N.; Salar, O.; Ollivere, B.J.; Forward, D.P.; Weerasuriya, N.; Moppett, I.K.; Moran, C.G. Evolution of the Hip Fracture Population: Time to Consider the Future? A Retrospective Observational Analysis. *BMJ Open* **2014**, *4*, e004405. [CrossRef] [PubMed]
4. Roche, J.J.W.; Wenn, R.T.; Sahota, O.; Moran, C.G. Effect of Comorbidities and Postoperative Complications on Mortality after Hip Fracture in Elderly People: Prospective Observational Cohort Study. *Br. Med. J.* **2005**, *331*, 1374–1376. [CrossRef] [PubMed]
5. Grigoryan, K.V.; Javedan, H.; Rudolph, J.L. Orthogeriatric Care Models and Outcomes in Hip Fracture Patients: A Systematic Review and Meta-Analysis. *J. Orthop. Trauma* **2014**, *28*, e49–e55. [CrossRef] [PubMed]
6. Patel, J.N.; Klein, D.S.; Sreekumar, S.; Liporace, F.A.; Yoon, R.S. Outcomes in Multidisciplinary Team-Based Approach in Geriatric Hip Fracture Care: A Systematic Review. *J. Am. Acad. Orthop. Surg.* **2020**, *28*, 128–133. [CrossRef] [PubMed]
7. Van Heghe, A.; Mordant, G.; Dupont, J.; Dejaeger, M.; Laurent, M.R.; Gielen, E. Effects of Orthogeriatric Care Models on Outcomes of Hip Fracture Patients: A Systematic Review and Meta-Analysis. *Calcif. Tissue Int.* **2022**, *110*, 162–184. [CrossRef] [PubMed]
8. Mangram, A.J.; Shifflette, V.K.; Mitchell, C.D.; Johnson, V.A.; Lorenzo, M.; Truitt, M.S.; Goel, A.; Lyons, M.; Dunn, E.L. The Creation of a Geriatric Trauma Unit "G-60". *Am. Surg.* **2011**, *77*, 1144–1146. [CrossRef] [PubMed]
9. Schuijt, H.J.; Kusen, J.; van Hernen, J.J.; van der Vet, P.; Geraghty, O.; Smeeing, D.P.J.; van der Velde, D. Orthogeriatric Trauma Unit Improves Patient Outcomes in Geriatric Hip Fracture Patients. *Geriatr. Orthop. Surg. Rehabil.* **2020**, *11*, 2151459320949476. [CrossRef] [PubMed]
10. Flikweert, E.R.; Wendt, K.W.; Diercks, R.L.; Izaks, G.J.; Stewart, R.; Stevens, M.; Reininga, I.H.F. A Comprehensive Multidisciplinary Care Pathway for Hip Fractures Better Outcome than Usual Care? *Injury* **2021**, *52*, 1819–1825. [CrossRef]
11. Campbell, H.; Hotchkiss, R.; Bradshaw, N.; Porteous, M. Integrated Care Pathways. *BMJ* **1998**, *316*, 133–137. [CrossRef] [PubMed]
12. Every, N.R.; Hochman, J.; Becker, R.; Kopecky, S.; Cannon, C.P. Critical Pathways: A Review. Committee on Acute Cardiac Care, Council on Clinical Cardiology, American Heart Association. *Circulation* **2000**, *101*, 461–465. [CrossRef] [PubMed]
13. Rotter, T.; Kinsman, L.; James, E.L.; Machotta, A.; Gothe, H.; Willis, J.; Snow, P.; Kugler, J. Clinical Pathways: Effects on Professional Practice, Patient Outcomes, Length of Stay and Hospital Costs. *Cochrane Database Syst. Rev.* **2010**, *3*, CD006632. [CrossRef] [PubMed]
14. Werner, M.; Macke, C.; Gogol, M.; Krettek, C.; Liodakis, E. Differences in Hip Fracture Care in Europe: A Systematic Review of Recent Annual Reports of Hip Fracture Registries. *Eur. J. Trauma Emerg. Surg.* **2022**, *48*, 1625–1638. [CrossRef] [PubMed]
15. Würdemann, F.S.; Krijnen, P.; van Zwet, E.W.; Arends, A.J.; Heetveld, M.J.; Trappenburg, M.C.; Hegeman, J.H.; Schipper, I.B.; Calf, A.H.; van Egmond, P.W.; et al. Trends in Data Quality and Quality Indicators 5 Years after Implementation of the Dutch Hip Fracture Audit. *Eur. J. Trauma Emerg. Surg.* **2022**, *48*, 4783–4796. [CrossRef] [PubMed]
16. Fox, F.; Drew, S.; Gregson, C.L.; Patel, R.; Chesser, T.J.S.; Johansen, A.; Javaid, M.K.; Griffin, X.L.; Gooberman-Hill, R. Complex Organisational Factors Influence Multidisciplinary Care for Patients with Hip Fractures: A Qualitative Study of Barriers and Facilitators to Service Delivery. *BMC Musculoskelet. Disord.* **2023**, *24*, 128. [CrossRef]
17. Suter, E.; Oelke, N.D.; Adair, C.E.; Armitage, G.D. Ten Key Principles for Successful Health Systems Integration. *Healthc. Q.* **2009**, *13*, 16–23. [CrossRef] [PubMed]
18. Evans-Lacko, S.; Jarrett, M.; McCrone, P.; Thornicroft, G. Facilitators and Barriers to Implementing Clinical Care Pathways. *BMC Health Serv. Res.* **2010**, *10*, 182. [CrossRef] [PubMed]
19. Latina, R.; Salomone, K.; D'angelo, D.; Coclite, D.; Castellini, G.; Gianola, S.; Fauci, A.; Napoletano, A.; Iacorossi, L.; Iannone, P. Towards a New System for the Assessment of the Quality in Care Pathways: An Overview of Systematic Reviews. *Int. J. Environ. Res. Public Health* **2020**, *17*, 8634. [CrossRef] [PubMed]
20. Kleinheksel, A.J.; Rockich-Winston, N.; Tawfik, H.; Wyatt, T.R. Demystifying Content Analysis. *Am. J. Pharm. Educ.* **2020**, *84*, 7113. [CrossRef]
21. Startpagina—Proximale Femurfracturen-Richtlijn-Richtlijnendatabase. Available online: https://richtlijnendatabase.nl/richtlijn/proximale_femurfracturen/proximale_femurfracturen_-_startpagina.html (accessed on 26 October 2022).

22. Moore, L.; Lavoie, A.; Bourgeois, G.; Lapointe, J. Donabedian's Structure-Process-Outcome Quality of Care Model: Validation in an Integrated Trauma System. *J. Trauma Acute Care Surg.* **2015**, *78*, 1168–1175. [CrossRef] [PubMed]
23. Fragility Fracture Network Orthogeriatric Care Model. Available online: https://fragilityfracturenetwork.org/wp-content/uploads/2023/10/ocm-2-pdf.pdf (accessed on 18 July 2023).
24. *To Err Is Human: Building a Safer Health System*; Kohn, L.T.; Corrigan, J.M.; Donaldson, M.S. (Eds.) National Academies Press (US): Washington, DC, USA, 2000; ISBN 0-309-06837-1.
25. Vanhaecht, K.; De Witte, K.; Depreitere, R.; Sermeus, W. Clinical Pathway Audit Tools: A Systematic Review. *J. Nurs. Manag.* **2006**, *14*, 529–537. [CrossRef] [PubMed]
26. Whittle, C. ICPAT: Integrated Care Pathways Appraisal Tool. *Int. J. Care Pathways* **2009**, *13*, 75–77. [CrossRef]
27. Whittle, C.L.; Mcdonald, P.S.; Dunn, L.; de Luc, K. Developing the Integrated Care Pathway Appraisal Tool (ICPAT): A Pilot Study. *Int. J. Care Pathways* **2004**, *8*, 77–81. [CrossRef]
28. Falaschi, P.; Marsh, D. *Orthogeriatrics: The Management of Older Patients with Fragility Fractures*, 2nd ed.; Springer: New York, NY, USA, 2021; ISBN 978-3-030-48125-4.
29. Panella, M.; Marchisio, S.; Di Stanislao, F. Reducing Clinical Variations with Clinical Pathways: Do Pathways Work? *Int. J. Qual. Health Care* **2003**, *15*, 509–521. [CrossRef] [PubMed]
30. Solberg, L.B.; Vesterhus, E.B.; Hestnes, I.; Ahmed, M.V.; Ommundsen, N.; Westberg, M.; Frihagen, F. Comparing Two Different Orthogeriatric Models of Care for Hip Fracture Patients: An Observational Prospective Cross-Sectional Study. *BMJ Open Qual.* **2023**, *12*, e002302. [CrossRef] [PubMed]
31. Kammerlander, C.; Roth, T.; Friedman, S.M.; Suhm, N.; Luger, T.J.; Kammerlander-Knauer, U.; Krappinger, D.; Blauth, M. Ortho-Geriatric Service-a Literature Review Comparing Different Models. *Osteoporos. Int.* **2010**, *21*, 637–646. [CrossRef]
32. van Bremen, H.E.; Seppala, L.J.; Gans, E.; Johannes, H.; van der Velde, N.; Willems, H.C. *Defining Optimal Orthogeriatric Hip Fracture Care: A Delphi Consensus Approach*; Amsterdam UMC: Amsterdam, The Netherlands, 2024; (*manuscript in preparation*).

Journal of
Clinical Medicine

MDPI

Article

Prognostic Factors for Mortality in Patients Aged 90 Years and Older with Proximal Femoral Fractures Undergoing Surgery: A Retrospective Study

Suguru Yokoo [1,2,*], Naofumi Shiota [1], Toru Sato [1], Sho Muguruma [1], Chuji Terada [2], Masanori Yorimitsu [3] and Toshifumi Ozaki [4]

1 Department of Orthopaedic Surgery, National Hospital Organization Okayama Medical Center, Okayama 701-1192, Japan; naofumi@mx1.tiki.ne.jp (N.S.); sato.toru.ez@mail.hosp.go.jp (T.S.); s.muguo1@gmail.com (S.M.)
2 Department of Orthopaedic Surgery, Fukuyama City Hospital, Hiroshima 721-8511, Japan; ccterada@yahoo.co.jp
3 Department of Musculoskeletal Traumatology, Faculty of Medicine, Dentistry, and Pharmaceutical Sciences, Okayama University, Okayama 700-8558, Japan; mayorimitsu@minos.ocn.ne.jp
4 Department of Orthopaedic Surgery, Okayama University Graduate School of Medicine, Dentistry, and Pharmaceutical Sciences, Okayama 700-8558, Japan; tozaki@md.okayama-u.ac.jp
* Correspondence: d04sm100@yahoo.co.jp; Tel.: +81-84-941-5151; Fax: +81-84-941-5159

Abstract: Background/Objectives: Proximal femoral fractures (PFFs) among individuals aged ≥90 years are becoming more common with an aging population and are associated with high morbidity and mortality. This study analyzed the prognostic factors influencing survival in nonagenarian patients undergoing surgery for PFFs. **Methods:** We enrolled 285 patients who underwent surgery between 2016 and 2022. Patients were classified into two groups: those with postoperative survival >1 year (L) and those with postoperative survival ≤1 year (D). Factors assessed included age, sex, body mass index (BMI), cognitive impairment, fracture type, surgical timing, length of hospital stay, implant type, preoperative hemoglobin/albumin/white blood cell levels, and Geriatric Nutritional Risk Index (GNRI). **Results:** The mean age at surgery was 93.2 ± 2.8 years (mean follow-up = 18.9 months). The 12-month mortality rate was 28.8%. Intertrochanteric fractures were observed in 136/47 patients, and femoral neck fractures were observed in 67/35 patients in the L/D group, respectively ($p = 0.13$). Days from admission to surgery were not significantly associated with mortality ($p = 0.56$). The mean hospital stay was 17/22 days in the L/D group, respectively. Univariate analysis identified age, BMI, cognitive impairment, albumin level, and GNRI as statistically significant predictors. Multivariate analysis revealed length of hospital stay (odds ratio [OR] = 1.048 [95% confidence interval (CI): 1.019–1.078]; $p = 0.001$), cognitive impairment (OR = 3.082 [95% CI: 1.367–6.945]; $p = 0.007$), and GNRI (OR = 0.929 [95% CI: 0.901–0.958]; $p < 0.001$) as independent predictors of mortality. **Conclusions:** This study identified cognitive impairment, a low GNRI, and prolonged hospital stay as independent prognostic factors for 1-year mortality in nonagenarian patients with PFFs. These findings highlight the importance of addressing malnutrition and cognitive decline through tailored interventions, alongside optimizing surgical timing and hospital care. A multidisciplinary approach remains essential for improving survival outcomes in this vulnerable population.

Keywords: body mass index; cognitive impairment; geriatric nutritional risk index; prognostic factor; proximal femoral fracture

1. Introduction

Proximal femoral fractures (PFFs) are prevalent among older adults and pose significant clinical challenges. With an aging society, the occurrence of PFFs among nonagenarians has become increasingly common. Japan is among the most rapidly aging countries globally, with >10% of its population aged ≥80 years [1,2]. As populations age, the incidence of PFFs is expected to increase [3,4]. Consequently, research on the prevention, treatment, and prognosis of PFFs is becoming increasingly important [5,6].

A previous study [7] found that individuals aged ≥85 years have a 15–18-fold higher risk of hip fracture than do those aged 50–54 years. Another study [8] reported that the incidence of PFFs among individuals aged ≥90 years is eight times higher than that among those in their seventies. Previous studies [9,10] have shown that PFFs are associated with high mortality rates and significant morbidity.

The risk of PFFs increases with age, primarily due to osteoporosis, making these fractures a significant cause of morbidity and mortality in advanced age [11]. Hip fractures profoundly impact the function and quality of life of patients aged ≥90 years. While surgical intervention and early rehabilitation remain the standard treatment for PFFs, limited data exist on surgical outcomes in nonagenarians, leaving many aspects of their prognosis unclear [12].

Multidisciplinary approaches play a crucial role in optimizing outcomes in older patients with hip fractures. Integrated orthogeriatric treatment models—involving surgeons, geriatricians, physiotherapists, and nutritionists—have been shown to reduce complications and improve mortality rates in older populations [13,14]. Given the unique physiological and psychological challenges faced by nonagenarians, including higher rates of comorbidities and complications, a collaborative approach tailored to their needs is essential for improving survival and recovery [13].

Mortality after hip fracture surgery is influenced by multiple factors, including age, time to surgery, sex, a high American Society of Anesthesiologists (ASA) score, cognitive impairment, and malnutrition [11,12,15]. Various scoring systems have been developed to predict postoperative outcomes in older patients with hip fractures. Among these, the Nottingham Hip Fracture Score is widely used to estimate the risk of mortality, particularly within the first 30 days after surgery. This score incorporates variables such as age, sex, preinjury mobility, and comorbidities to provide a comprehensive assessment of patient risk [16].

Nutritional status, as assessed using tools such as the Geriatric Nutritional Risk Index (GNRI) and cognitive impairment are particularly critical determinants of postoperative outcomes in older populations. The GNRI provides a comprehensive evaluation of nutritional status by incorporating both serum albumin levels and body mass index (BMI), which are independently associated with mortality in older adults with hip fractures. Recent studies, including a meta-analysis, have validated the predictive value of the GNRI for postoperative complications, highlighting its potential as a reliable prognostic tool [17]. Similarly, cognitive impairment is a well-recognized risk factor for poor surgical outcomes, including increased mortality and reduced functional recovery. A recent systematic review has revealed that dementia significantly contributes to early mortality after hip fracture surgery, although it primarily focused on younger older adult populations overall [15]. While prior studies have examined hip fracture outcomes in nonagenarians, many lacked using standardized cognitive scoring methods, which may underestimate the true impact of cognitive impairment [13]. The use of validated tools, such as the Abbreviated Mental Test Score (AMTS), provides a more objective and reliable assessment of cognitive status, enabling a clearer understanding of its influence on mortality.

Most existing studies on hip fractures in nonagenarians have focused on short-term outcomes, such as 30- or 90-day mortality, with limited attention to longer-term survival rates [18–20]. For example, while several studies have highlighted the immediate risks associated with surgery, few have systematically evaluated 1-year survival rates or the factors influencing them. Furthermore, while 1-year mortality data are relatively abundant for younger older populations, such as those in their seventies or eighties, these data are scarce for nonagenarians. Given the unique vulnerabilities of this age group, understanding 1-year outcomes is critical for guiding treatment strategies and improving prognostic predictions. We conducted this study to fill this gap by analyzing the 1-year survival outcomes and their associated prognostic factors in nonagenarian patients with PFFs.

Despite the identification of these risk factors, a consensus on the most predictive factors of mortality in patients aged ≥90 years with PFFs remains elusive. In this study, we aimed to analyze the surgical outcomes for PFFs in patients aged ≥90 years and to identify factors associated with their survival.

2. Materials and Methods

2.1. Ethics

The study was conducted in accordance with the Declaration of Helsinki and approved by the Institutional Review Board of the National Hospital Organization Okayama Medical Center (approval number: 2022-154; approval date: 20 December 2022). Informed consent was obtained from all subjects involved in the study.

2.2. Study Design and Participants

A total of 305 consecutive patients aged ≥90 years who underwent surgery for PFFs at our hospital between January 2016 and December 2022 were retrospectively reviewed. After excluding 20 patients because of insufficient follow-up, 285 patients were included in the study. Patients with postoperative survival >1 year were categorized as the L group, while those with postoperative survival ≤1 year were categorized as the D group. The exclusion criteria included fractures related to bone tumors and patients who had undergone osteosynthesis revision.

2.3. Operative Procedure

All patients underwent surgery under spinal or general anesthesia. Intertrochanteric fractures were treated using a Dynamic Hip System (DePuySynthes, Warsaw, IN, USA) or an intertrochanteric nail. The intertrochanteric nails used were the TFN-ADVANCED™ Proximal Femoral Nailing System (DePuySynthes) or the Unicorn nail (HOYA Technosurgical, Tokyo, Japan). The choice of implant was based on patient factors such as bone quality, fracture stability, and overall health status. Non-displaced femoral neck fractures were treated with cannulated cancellous hip screws, while displaced femoral neck fractures were managed with hemiarthroplasty. All patients were allowed full weight-bearing ambulation postoperatively.

2.4. Follow-Up

Hospital transfer was typically scheduled for approximately 14 days postoperatively, depending on patient progress. After transfer, patients were monitored at the outpatient clinic at 12 weeks, 6 months, 12 months, and annually thereafter—or until death. Survival status was ascertained through hospital follow-up visits or by contacting patients and their families. Mortality at 6 months, 12 months, and at the end of the study period was documented. Patients who survived were followed up for ≥12 months, while those who passed away were followed up until the date of death, which marked the endpoint for mortality analysis. Thus, the follow-up duration ranged from the date of surgery to death or the conclusion of the study. The primary endpoint was either death or the conclusion of the study (December 2023).

2.5. Determination of Prognostic Risk Factors

Factors evaluated included age; sex; BMI; cognitive impairment; fracture type; days from injury to surgery; days from admission to surgery; length of hospital stay; duration of surgery; levels of hemoglobin, albumin, and white blood cells; and Geriatric Nutritional Risk Index (GNRI) on admission. The GNRI was calculated based on serum albumin levels and body weight relative to ideal body weight using the following equation:

$$\text{GNRI} = (1.489 \times \text{serum albumin (g/dL)}) + (41.7 \times \text{actual body weight (kg)/ideal body weight (kg)}) \quad (1)$$

where ideal body weight was defined as the weight corresponding to a BMI of 22 kg/m^2. This index is commonly used to assess nutritional risk in older patients [21]. Data were collected by reviewing hospital records and interviewing patients and their relatives. Cognitive impairment was assessed using the AMTS, with a threshold of 7 points (with scores of $\leq$6 indicating impairment). Prefracture functional status was assessed and categorized into five groups based on the degree of mobility: patients who could walk independently without assistive devices (Free Walk), those who required a cane (Cane Gait), those using a walker (Walker), and those who were either wheelchair-bound (Wheelchair) or bedridden (Bedridden). For further analysis, these categories were consolidated into two groups: those who were able to walk (Free Walk, Cane Gait, or Walker) and those who were unable to walk (Wheelchair or Bedridden).

2.6. Statistical Analysis

Differences in patient characteristics were assessed using the chi-square test for categorical variables and the unpaired *t*-test for continuous variables. Post hoc power analysis was conducted following the univariate analysis to ensure that the study had sufficient statistical power to detect significant differences, with a threshold set to 0.80. Multivariate analysis was subsequently performed using logistic regression to identify independent factors associated with mortality. Receiver Operating Characteristic (ROC) curve analysis was employed to determine the optimal cut-off values for statistically significant variables in the univariate or multivariate analyses. The Youden index was calculated to identify cut-off values that maximized the balance between sensitivity and specificity, and the area under the curve (AUC) was used to assess predictive accuracy. Patient survival was analyzed using the Kaplan–Meier method, and between-group differences in survival were assessed using the log-rank test. Statistical significance was set at $p < 0.05$. All statistical analyses were conducted using GraphPad Prism (version 8.0; GraphPad Software, San Diego, CA, USA).

3. Results

The mean age at surgery was 93.2 ± 2.8 years. The mean follow-up period was 18.9 (range = 0–80) months (Table 1). The cohort comprised 43 males and 242 females. The numbers of deaths within 1 month, 6 months, and 12 months after surgery were 4 (1.4%), 54 (18.9%), and 82 (28.8%), respectively. According to the Kaplan–Meier method, the median survival time was 37 months (Figure 1). The survival probability declined steeply during the first year after surgery, with mortality rates of 1.4%, 18.9%, and 28.8% at 1 month, 6 months, and 12 months, respectively.

Table 1. Patient characteristics.

Characteristic	Value
Age, years	93.2 ± 2.8
Sex	
Female	242
Male	43
Fracture type	
Trochanter	183
Neck	102
Treatment	
Compression hip screw	94
Nail	89
Hemiarthroplasty	74
Cannulated cancellous hip screws	28
Days from injury to surgery	3.0 ± 4.0
Days from admission to surgery	1.9 ± 2.6
Length of hospital stay (days)	18.9 ± 9.3
Follow-up period (months)	18.2 ± 15.4

Data are presented as *n* or mean ± SD.

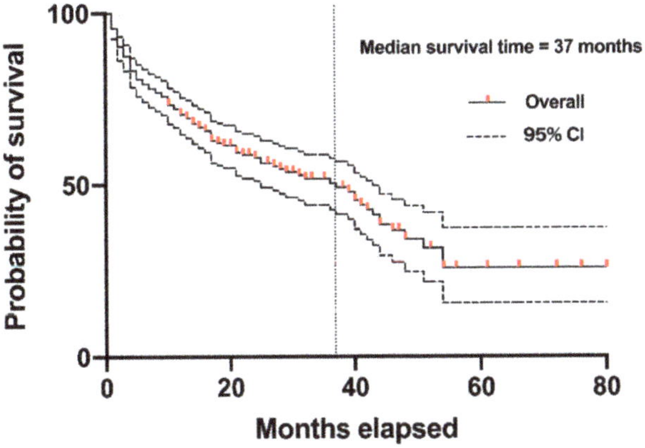

Figure 1. Kaplan–Meier curve for overall survival illustrating the probability of survival following surgical intervention for proximal femoral fractures. The solid line represents the Kaplan–Meier curve. The dashed lines represent the 95% confidence intervals. The median survival time was 37 months, with a 95% confidence interval ranging from 29.0 to 44.5 months. The mortality rates were 1.4% (n = 4), 18.9% (n = 54), and 28.8% (n = 82) at 1 month, 6 months, and 12 months after surgery, respectively. The curve represents long-term survival outcomes up to approximately 8 years.

A total of 183 patients had intertrochanteric fractures; 102 had femoral neck fractures (Table 2). Among the patients with intertrochanteric fractures, 94 and 84 were treated with the Dynamic Hip System and intertrochanteric nails, respectively. Among the patients with femoral neck fractures, 28 were treated with cannulated cancellous hip screws, while 74 underwent hemiarthroplasty. The L group (patients who survived >12 months after surgery) included 136 and 67 patients with intertrochanteric and femoral neck fractures, respectively. The D group (patients who died within 12 months after surgery) included 47 and 35 patients with intertrochanteric and femoral neck fractures, respectively (p = 0.13).

Table 2. Univariate analysis of factors affecting survival.

Variables	Alive (n = 203)	Deceased (n = 82)	p-Value
Age, years	92.8 ± 2.6	94.0 ± 3.1	0.015
Sex			0.10
Female	177	65	
Male	26	17	
BMI, kg/m²	20.2 ± 2.8	18.7 ± 3.3	<0.0001
Cognitive impairment			0.0004
Yes	141	73	
No	62	9	
Fracture type			0.13
Trochanter	136	47	
Neck	67	35	
Implant type			
Dynamic Hip System	69	25	0.48
Intertrochanteric nail	67	22	
Cannulated cancellous hip screws	18	10	
Hemiarthroplasty	49	25	
Days from injury to surgery	3.1 ± 4.2	2.7 ± 3.5	0.50
Days from admission to surgery	2.0 ± 2.7	1.9 ± 2.4	0.56
Length of hospital stay (days)	17 ± 7.8	22 ± 11.7	0.003
Duration of surgery (minutes)	82 ± 29.7	80 ± 26.1	0.77
Hemoglobin	10.8 ± 1.7	10.7 ± 1.9	0.51
Albumin	3.6 ± 0.46	3.3 ± 0.51	<0.0001
White blood cells	9.1 ± 3.3	9.0 ± 3.9	0.62
GNRI	91.8 ± 9.1	84.9 ± 10.2	<0.0001

Data are presented as n or mean ± SD. GNRI: Geriatric Nutritional Risk Index.

The mean surgical duration was 82.3 ± 29.7 min for the L group and 80.2 ± 26.1 min for the D group (p = 0.77). The mean duration from injury to surgery was 3.0 ± 4.0 days; the mean duration from admission to surgery was 1.9 ± 2.6 days; and the mean length of hospital stay was 18.9 ± 9.3 days. The mean durations from injury to surgery were 3.1 ± 4.2 and 2.7 ± 3.5 days in the L and D groups, respectively (p = 0.50). The mean durations from admission to surgery were 2.0 ± 2.7 and 1.9 ± 2.4 days in the L and D groups, respectively (p = 0.56). The mean lengths of hospital stay were 17 ± 7.8 and 22 ± 11.7 days in the L and D groups, respectively (p = 0.003) (Table 2).

3.1. Univariate Analysis of Prognostic Factors

Other examined variables included age (mean = 92.8 years in the L group and 94.0 years in the D group; p = 0.015); sex (male/female = 26/177 in the L group and 17/65 in the D group; p = 0.10); BMI (mean = 20.2 kg/m^2 in the L group and 18.7 kg/m^2 in the D group; $p < 0.0001$); cognitive impairment (69.5% in the L group and 89.0% in the D group; p = 0.0004); prefracture functional status (ambulatory patients = 86.2% in the L group and 81.7% in the D group; p = 0.2261); hemoglobin level on admission (mean = 10.8 g/dL in the L group and 10.7 g/dL in the D group; p = 0.51); albumin level on admission (mean = 3.6 g/dL in the L group and 3.3 g/dL in the D group; $p < 0.0001$); white blood cell count (mean = 9.1 µL in the L group and 9.0 µL in the D group; p = 0.62); GNRI on admission (mean = 91.8 in the L group and 84.9 in the D group; $p < 0.0001$); and implant type (Dynamic Hip System/intertrochanteric nail/cannulated cancellous hip screws/hemiarthroplasty = 69/67/18/49 in the L group and 25/22/10/25 in the D group; p = 0.48) (Table 2). In the univariate analysis, age, BMI, length of hospital stay, cognitive impairment, albumin level on admission, and GNRI were found to be significantly associated with overall survival. Post hoc power analyses were conducted to confirm the adequacy of the sample size for these key variables. The power achieved for each variable was as follows: age (0.7661), BMI (0.9826), length of hospital stay (0.9156), cognitive impairment (0.9858), albumin level (0.982), and GNRI (0.9998). The results demonstrated sufficient statistical power for most variables, except for age, which had a slightly lower but still acceptable power.

3.2. Multivariate Analysis of Prognostic Factors

Multivariate analysis demonstrated that the length of hospital stay (odds ratio [OR] = 1.048 [95% confidence interval (CI): 1.019–1.078]; p = 0.001), cognitive impairment (OR = 3.082 [95% CI: 1.367–6.945]; p = 0.007), and GNRI (OR = 0.929 [95% CI: 0.901–0.958]; $p < 0.001$) were independently associated with mortality (Table 3).

Table 3. Multivariate analysis of factors affecting survival.

Variables	OR	Interval		p-Value
		Lower	Upper	
Length of hospital stay	1.05	1.02	1.08	0.001
Cognitive impairment	3.08	1.37	6.95	0.007
GNRI	0.93	0.90	0.96	<0.001

GNRI: Geriatric Nutritional Risk Index.

Although the age, BMI, and albumin level variables were statistically significant in the univariate analysis, they were not retained in the final multivariate model following stepwise selection. This was attributed to their relatively small independent effects compared to other variables, such as the length of hospital stay, cognitive impairment, and GNRI, which were retained in the final multivariate model.

3.3. Kaplan–Meier Survival Analysis

Kaplan–Meier survival analysis was conducted to further explore the impact of the GNRI and cognitive impairment on patient survival. The GNRI cut-off value was determined using the ROC curve, which evaluates the diagnostic ability of the GNRI to predict survival outcomes. The area under the curve (AUC) was 0.68 (95% CI: 0.61–0.754, indicating moderate predictive accuracy. A Youden index cut-off value of 83.72 was established to optimally differentiate between higher- and lower-risk patients (Figure 2). This threshold reflects a balance between sensitivity and specificity, supporting its clinical utility in identifying patients at an elevated risk of poor outcomes.

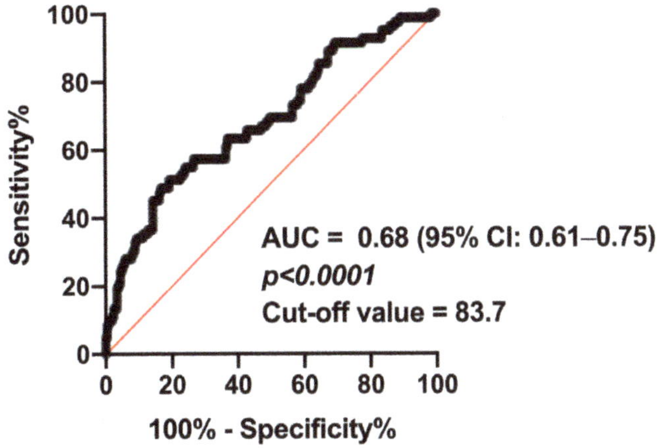

Figure 2. Receiver operating characteristic curve based on a sample size of 285 patients illustrating the diagnostic ability of the Geriatric Nutritional Risk Index in predicting survival outcomes. The area under the curve (AUC) was 0.68 (95% confidence interval [CI]: 0.61–0.75) ($p < 0.0001$). The Youden index cut-off value was 83.7.

Additionally, patients were grouped based on cognitive impairment, which was defined by an AMTS score of 7. The Kaplan–Meier survival curves indicated that patients without cognitive impairment had a significantly higher survival probability than did those with cognitive impairment ($p = 0.01$; log-rank test) (Figure 3b).

(a)

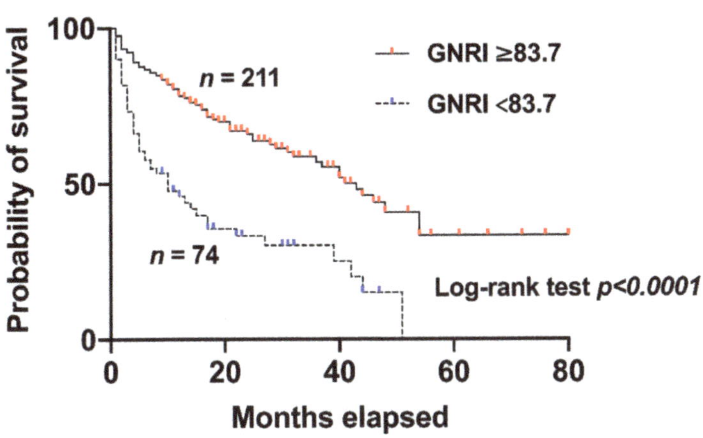

Figure 3. *Cont.*

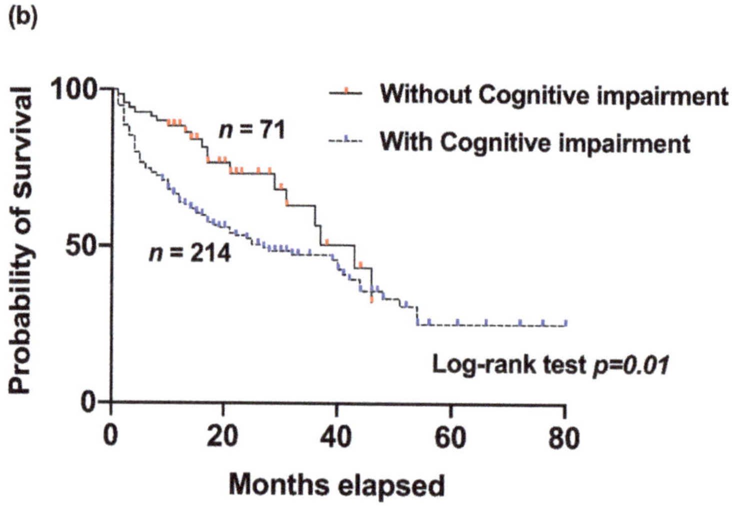

Figure 3. Kaplan–Meier survival curves for Geriatric Nutritional Risk Index (GNRI) and cognitive impairment: (**a**) Kaplan–Meier survival curves comparing patients with a higher (≥83.7) and lower (<83.72) GNRI. The survival probability is shown over the elapsed months, indicating that patients with a higher GNRI were found to have significantly better survival outcomes ($p < 0.0001$; log-rank test). (**b**) Kaplan–Meier survival curves comparing patients with and without cognitive impairment (defined as an Abbreviated Mental Test Score of 7). The analysis shows that patients without cognitive impairment were found to have significantly better survival outcomes compared to those with cognitive impairment ($p = 0.01$; log-rank test).

4. Discussion

4.1. Key Prognostic Factors for Survival

This study identified several prognostic factors for survival in patients aged ≥90 years with PFFs, including BMI, cognitive impairment, albumin level, and GNRI. These findings highlight the importance of nutritional and cognitive assessments in this vulnerable population. The high post hoc power achieved for the key prognostic factors (age, BMI, cognitive impairment, albumin level, and GNRI) supports the reliability of the study's findings. The powers for BMI, cognitive impairment, albumin level, and GNRI were all >0.98, indicating that the sample size was sufficient to detect significant differences in survival outcomes. Although the power for age was slightly lower at 0.7661, it was still within the acceptable limits for drawing conclusions.

4.2. Mortality and Hospital Stay

In this study, longer hospital stays, a lower BMI on admission, cognitive impairment, and lower albumin levels on admission were associated with higher mortality rates. Ko et al. [22] have reported that shorter hospital stays for older patients with hip fractures could be feasible without adversely affecting outcomes provided that tailored postoperative care has been implemented. Early surgery and rehabilitation are crucial for reducing mortality rates, whereas the length of hospital stay directly affects prognosis [9]. However, it is important to note that the length of hospital stay is influenced by institutional policies, social factors, and logistical constraints, including the availability of rehabilitation hospitals, which is particularly relevant in Japan where postoperative transfers are common. These factors may not directly reflect the patient's clinical outcomes, highlighting the need to evaluate the length of hospital stay alongside other variables when assessing mortality risk.

4.3. Nutritional Status: GNRI, BMI, and the Obesity Paradox

Previous studies [10,15] have also demonstrated that both a low BMI and low serum albumin levels are independently associated with higher mortality rates in patients with PFFs. Given that the GNRI combines these two critical indicators of nutritional status, it provides a more comprehensive assessment of malnutrition and its impact on survival outcomes. However, to our knowledge, no previous studies have specifically examined the GNRI as a prognostic factor in nonagenarians with hip fractures. Our study is the first to demonstrate that a low GNRI is significantly associated with increased mortality in patients aged ≥90 years, highlighting the importance of addressing nutritional status in this highly vulnerable population. Our findings suggest that, similar to younger cohorts, malnutrition remains a critical determinant of survival, and interventions aimed at improving nutritional status could play a key role in improving outcomes for nonagenarians with hip fractures. Older patients with cognitive impairment have poorer outcomes after hip fracture surgery, including higher mortality rates and reduced functional recovery [23,24]. A multidisciplinary approach is essential for managing patients with dementia undergoing hip fracture surgery, focusing on tailored postoperative care to improve outcomes.

Hypoalbuminemia (low serum albumin levels) has been found to significantly increase postoperative complications, including infections, delayed wound healing, and prolonged hospital stays [25]. Preoperative nutritional status is crucial for determining patient outcomes, highlighting the importance of appropriate nutritional management and postoperative care strategies. Lower preoperative serum albumin levels are associated with higher postoperative mortality and morbidity rates [26,27]. Routine assessment of albumin levels as part of the preoperative evaluation could enhance long-term survival outcomes in this vulnerable patient population.

Previous studies have shown that a high BMI is associated with increased morbidity and mortality rates among older patients with PFFs. For instance, Soliman et al. [28] have highlighted higher rates of comorbidities and post-trauma complications in patients with obesity than in those with a normal weight. Similarly, another study [12] has emphasized the negative impact of a high BMI on patient outcomes owing to the increased risk of complications. However, the findings of the present study suggest that, in patients aged ≥90 years, a high BMI may be linked to better survival outcomes. This could be because of a better nutritional status and greater muscle mass, which are crucial for recovery in very old individuals. This "obesity paradox" indicates that a high BMI may provide a survival advantage in this age group by offering greater energy reserves during acute illness or injury. In contrast, a low BMI has been consistently associated with poorer surgical outcomes, including a higher postoperative mortality rate, delayed recovery, and an increased risk of complications. A low BMI often reflects malnutrition and sarcopenia, conditions that compromise the body's ability to heal and recover after major trauma or surgery [29,30]. Malnutrition, in particular, has been linked to immune dysfunction, prolonged wound healing, and an increased susceptibility to infections, all of which can significantly impair recovery after hip fracture surgery. This highlights the importance of early nutritional assessment and intervention, especially in the oldest old population. Additionally, other studies [31,32] have indicated that a high BMI in later life may be associated with a lower risk of mortality from certain conditions, particularly cardiovascular disease. Individuals who entered adulthood with a normal BMI and gradually became overweight tended to live the longest [33]. These findings highlight the need for personalized medical approaches in treating very old patients with PFFs. While traditionally viewed as a negative factor, a high BMI might be beneficial for the oldest old, suggesting that clinical guidelines should be refined to account for these unique characteristics. Further research is needed to fully understand this association and its implications for patient care.

4.4. Surgical Timing and Patient-Specific Factors

Early surgery is expected to reduce mortality rates, enhance functional recovery, and decrease the risk of complications in patients with PFFs [34,35]. However, acute medical conditions, such as heart failure, pneumonia, severe coagulation disorders, and metabolic abnormalities, may contraindicate early surgery [12,36,37]. Stabilizing the overall condition of older patients with lower surgical tolerance before proceeding may be necessary. In the present study, the number of days from admission to surgery was not significantly associated with mortality ($p = 0.56$). This finding contrasts with those of previous studies suggesting that early surgery improves outcomes in patients with hip fractures [34,35]. One possible explanation for this discrepancy is that the relatively short time from admission to surgery (mean 2.0 days) in our cohort may have limited the ability to detect significant differences. Additionally, many patients experienced delays due to referral processes prior to hospital admission, which may have influenced the definition of "delayed surgery" compared to other studies. This highlights the importance of evaluating pre-hospital factors that could impact surgical timing and outcomes.

Furthermore, the lack of a significant association between implant type and survival outcomes aligns with the notion that patient-specific factors, such as nutritional status and comorbidities, play a more critical role in determining survival than does implant selection.

4.5. Mortality Trends and Prognostic Insights

While many reports have focused on the prognosis of patients with PFFs, few have specifically addressed patients aged >90 years. Previous studies [38–41] have indicated that the 1-year mortality rate for surgically treated patients aged >90 years ranges from 12.1% to 54.7%. In the present study, the 1-year mortality rate was 28.8%, which is consistent with these findings. Poor prognostic factors in the surgical management of PFFs in patients aged ≥90 years include a preoperative ASA score of 4, female sex, delayed surgery, and pre-existing heart disease and endocrinopathies. In the present study, no patients with an ASA score of 4 underwent surgery. Although no significant difference was found regarding sex, a trend toward higher mortality rates among males was observed. Generally, the mortality rate after PFFs is higher among men than women [42–44]. This may be partly explained by the generally shorter life expectancy among men [45].

Non-surgical management of PFFs in older individuals with frailty is associated with higher mortality rates [46]. Surgery for femoral neck fractures in patients aged >90 years significantly was found to improve survival rates compared to non-surgical treatment [47]. Timely surgery and proper preoperative management can significantly improve outcomes and reduce mortality in this population [11,48].

4.6. Study Strengths and Limitations

This study has several strengths. First, the treatment outcomes were derived from a single-center study, which ensured consistent treatment protocols, minimized potential biases often associated with multicenter studies, and allowed for homogeneity in surgical teams and postoperative care. This consistency has likely enhanced the internal validity of our findings. Second, this study included a large sample size of 285 patients aged ≥90 years with PFFs, which represent a patient demographic that is typically underrepresented in the existing literature. Lastly, the high follow-up rate of 93.4% (285/305 patients) minimizes the risk of follow-up bias and reinforces the robustness of the study's findings.

The main limitations of this study include its retrospective design and potential bias in data collection. As a retrospective study, it is subject to inherent biases, such as selection bias and information bias, which may affect the accuracy of the results. The retrospective nature of this study also limits our ability to establish causal relationships between the identified prognostic factors and mortality outcomes. Although multivariate analysis was used to adjust for confounding factors, residual confounding cannot be completely ruled out. While the sample size is large for this specific age group, it remains limited compared to studies with a broader population, potentially affecting the generalizability of the results. In this study, diabetes and cognitive impairment were selected as the primary comorbidities for analysis, as these conditions have been identified in prior studies as key prognostic factors. However, other comorbidities, such as cardiovascular and renal diseases, were excluded owing to data limitations and the need to maintain statistical power. Similarly, ASA scores were not included in this study, as specific documentation regarding ASA classifications was unavailable retrospectively from the medical records. Retrospectively assigning ASA scores based on subjective judgments, particularly for borderline categories such as ASA 2–3, posed a substantial risk of bias. This limitation highlights the necessity for standardized and systematic recording of ASA scores in future research to ensure more rigorous and reliable prognostic evaluations. This limitation may restrict the generalizability of our findings. Future studies should include a broader range of comorbidities to provide a more comprehensive analysis. Variations in treatment protocols across different healthcare facilities could lead to inconsistencies in patient care and outcomes. Moreover, while the single-center design ensures consistency, it may limit the generalizability of the findings to other healthcare settings with varying resources and treatment protocols. The focus on 1-year mortality may not capture long-term outcomes, and socioeconomic factors influencing patient outcomes may not have been adequately addressed. Despite these limitations, this study provides valuable insights into the mortality rates among nonagenarians following hip fracture surgery, contributing to the growing body of knowledge in geriatric orthopedics.

4.7. Future Research Directions

Future research should focus on validating the GNRI as a dynamic prognostic tool in nonagenarian patients with PFFs. While our study demonstrated its utility upon admission, it remains unclear whether the GNRI changes over the course of hospitalization and whether such changes correlate with clinical outcomes. Prospective studies should evaluate the impact of nutritional interventions on GNRI values and investigate whether improvements in GNRI are associated with better survival and functional recovery. Additionally, determining the optimal timing for GNRI assessment—whether at admission, postoperatively, or during rehabilitation—could enhance its clinical applicability. Such investigations could provide a clearer understanding of how to integrate the GNRI into routine clinical practice to improve outcomes in this vulnerable population. These future studies could address some of the limitations discussed in the following section, particularly regarding the retrospective design and limited assessment of comorbidities.

5. Conclusions

This study underscores the importance of identifying and managing specific prognostic factors in nonagenarian patients with PFFs. A low BMI, cognitive impairment, low albumin levels, and lengthy hospital stays were significantly associated with increased mortality rates. By addressing these factors through tailored clinical interventions, healthcare providers can improve the overall survival and quality of care for this vulnerable patient population. These findings highlight the need for a comprehensive multidisciplinary approach to treating older patients with hip fractures. Our study results suggest avenues for further research, including large-scale multicenter studies for generalization, long-term follow-up for deeper prognostic insights, and interventional studies, to improve treatment protocols.

Author Contributions: Conceptualization, S.Y.; Methodology, S.Y.; Validation, S.Y. and S.M.; Formal Analysis, S.Y.; Investigation, S.Y.; Resources, N.S. and T.S.; Data Curation, S.Y. and S.M.; Writing—Original Draft Preparation, S.Y.; Writing—Review and Editing, S.Y., N.S., T.S., S.M., C.T., M.Y. and T.O.; Visualization, S.Y.; Supervision, N.S.; Project Administration, S.Y. and N.S. All authors have read and agreed to the published version of the manuscript.

Funding: This research received no external funding.

Institutional Review Board Statement: The study was conducted in accordance with the Declaration of Helsinki and approved by the Institutional Review Board of the National Hospital Organization Okayama Medical Center (approval number: 2022-154; approval date: 20 December 2022).

Informed Consent Statement: Informed consent was obtained from all subjects involved in the study.

Data Availability Statement: Due to ethical considerations, we are unable to make the full dataset publicly available. However, we are open to discussing requests for anonymized data from qualified researchers under appropriate agreements.

Acknowledgments: The authors would like to acknowledge our institution for their contributions to the study, including support with patient data collection and surgical expertise.

Conflicts of Interest: The authors declare no conflicts of interest.

References

1. World Population Prospects 2022: Summary of Results. Available online: https://www.un.org/development/desa/pd/ (accessed on 19 July 2024).
2. Ageing and Health. Available online: https://www.who.int/news-room/fact-sheets/detail/ageing-and-health (accessed on 19 July 2024).
3. Stevens, J.A.; Rudd, R.A. The impact of decreasing U.S. hip fracture rates on future hip fracture estimates. *Osteoporos. Int.* **2013**, *24*, 2725–2728. [CrossRef] [PubMed]
4. Sing, C.W.; Lin, T.C.; Bartholomew, S.; Bell, J.S.; Bennett, C.; Beyene, K.; Bosco-Lévy, P.; Chan, A.H.Y.; Chandran, M.; Cheung, C.L.; et al. Global epidemiology of hip fractures: A study protocol using a common analytical platform among multiple countries. *BMJ Open* **2021**, *11*, e047258. [CrossRef] [PubMed]
5. Burge, R.; Dawson-Hughes, B.; Solomon, D.H.; Wong, J.B.; King, A.; Tosteson, A. Incidence and economic burden of osteoporosis-related fractures in the United States, 2005-2025. *J. Bone Miner. Res.* **2007**, *22*, 465–475. [CrossRef] [PubMed]
6. Walter, N.; Szymski, D.; Kurtz, S.; Alt, V.; Lowenberg, D.W.; Lau, E.; Rupp, M. Factors associated with mortality after proximal femoral fracture. *J. Orthop. Surg. Res.* **2023**, *24*, 31. [CrossRef]
7. Kang, H.Y.; Yang, K.H.; Kim, Y.N.; Moon, S.H.; Choi, W.J.; Kang, D.R.; Park, S.E. Incidence and mortality of hip fracture among the elderly population in South Korea: A population-based study using the national health insurance claims data. *BMC Public Health* **2010**, *10*, 230. [CrossRef] [PubMed]
8. Orimo, H.; Yaegashi, Y.; Onoda, T.; Fukushima, Y.; Hosoi, T.; Sakata, K. Hip fracture incidence in Japan: Estimates of new patients in 2007 and 20-year trends. *Arch. Osteoporos.* **2009**, *4*, 71–77. [CrossRef]
9. Aprato, A.; Bechis, M.; Buzzone, M.; Bistolfi, A.; Daghino, W.; Massè, A. No rest for elderly femur fracture patients: Early surgery and early ambulation decrease mortality. *J. Orthop. Traumatol.* **2020**, *21*, 12. [CrossRef]
10. Marom, O.; Paz, I.; Segal, D.; Topaz, G.; Abelson, N.; Tavdi, A.; Behrbalk, R.; Palmanovich, E.; Ohana, N.; Yaacobi, E. Proximal femur fractures in the elderly—A novel modality to predict mortality: The neutrophil-to-lymphocyte ratio. *J. Clin. Med.* **2023**, *12*, 456. [CrossRef]
11. Postler, A.; Posten, C.; Schubert, M.; Beyer, F.; Lützner, J.; Vicent, O.; Kleber, C.; Goronzy, J.; Kamin, K. Patients risk for mortality at 90 days after proximal femur fracture—A retrospective study in a tertiary care hospital. *BMC Geriatr.* **2024**, *24*, 130. [CrossRef]
12. Fischer, H.; Maleitzke, T.; Eder, C.; Ahmad, S.; Stöckle, U.; Braun, K.F. Management of proximal femur fractures in the elderly: Current concepts and treatment options. *Eur. J. Med. Res.* **2021**, *26*, 86. [CrossRef]
13. de Groot, R.; Nijmeijer, W.S.; Folbert, E.C.; Vollenbroek-Hutten, M.M.R.; Hegeman, J.H. 'Nonagenarians' with a hip fracture: Is a different orthogeriatric treatment strategy necessary? *Arch. Osteoporos.* **2020**, *15*, 19. [CrossRef] [PubMed]
14. Gialanella, B.; Santoro, R.; Prometti, P.; Giordano, A.; Monguzzi, V.; Comini, L.; Olivares, A.; Grioni, G. Functional recovery in hip fracture patients: The role of pharmacotherapy. *Aging Clin. Exp. Res.* **2020**, *32*, 49–57. [CrossRef] [PubMed]
15. Bui, M.; Nijmeijer, W.S.; Hegeman, J.H.; Witteveen, A.; Groothuis-Oudshoorn, C.G.M. Systematic review and meta-analysis of preoperative predictors for early mortality following hip fracture surgery. *Osteoporos. Int.* **2024**, *35*, 561–574. [CrossRef] [PubMed]
16. Maxwell, M.J.; Moran, C.G.; Moppett, I.K. Development and validation of a preoperative scoring system to predict 30 day mortality in patients undergoing hip fracture surgery. *Br. J. Anaesth.* **2008**, *101*, 511–517. [CrossRef] [PubMed]
17. Liu, W.; Li, M.; Lian, S.; Hou, X.; Ling, Y. Geriatric nutritional risk index as a predictor for postoperative complications in patients with solid cancers: A meta-analysis. *Front. Oncol.* **2024**, *14*, 1266291. [CrossRef]
18. Manoli, A., 3rd; Driesman, A.; Marwin, R.A.; Konda, S.; Leucht, P.; Egol, K.A. Short-term outcomes following hip fractures in patients at least 100 years old. *J. Bone Jt. Surg. Am.* **2017**, *99*, e68. [CrossRef]
19. Mayordomo-Cava, J.; Abásolo, L.; Montero-Fernandez, N.; Ortiz-Alonso, J.; Vidán-Astiz, M.; Serra-Rexach, J.A. Hip fracture in nonagenarians: Characteristics and factors related to 30-day mortality in 1177 patients. *J. Arthroplasty* **2020**, *35*, 1186–1193. [CrossRef]
20. Kadowaki, M.; Kono, M.; Nishiguchi, K.; Kakimaru, H.; Uchio, Y. Mortality in patients with hip fracture aged over 90 years: A report from a progressively aging island. *Arch. Gerontol. Geriatr.* **2012**, *54*, e113–e117. [CrossRef]
21. Bouillanne, O.; Morineau, G.; Dupont, C.; Coulombel, I.; Vincent, J.P.; Nicolis, I.; Benazeth, S.; Cynober, L.; Aussel, C. Geriatric Nutritional Risk Index: A new index for evaluating at-risk elderly medical patients. *Am. J. Clin. Nutr.* **2005**, *82*, 777–783. [CrossRef]
22. Ko, Y.S.; Kang, S.Y.; Lee, H.J.; Kim, H.S.; Yoo, J.J. Trends in hospital stay, complication rate, and mortality in hip fracture patients: A two-decade comparison at a national tertiary referral center. *J. Clin. Med.* **2024**, *13*, 3666. [CrossRef]

23. Intiso, D.; Di Rienzo, F.; Grimaldi, G.; Lombardi, T.; Fiore, P.; Maruzzi, G.; Iarossi, A.; Tolfa, M.; Pazienza, L. Survival and functional outcome in patients 90 years of age or older after hip fracture. *Age Ageing* **2009**, *38*, 619–622. [CrossRef] [PubMed]
24. Hou, M.; Zhang, Y.; Chen, A.C.; Liu, T.; Yang, H.; Zhu, X.; He, F. The effects of dementia on the prognosis and mortality of hip fracture surgery: A systematic review and meta-analysis. *Aging Clin. Exp. Res.* **2021**, *33*, 3161–3172. [CrossRef] [PubMed]
25. Residori, L.; Bortolami, O.; Di Francesco, V. Hypoalbuminemia increases complications in elderly patients operated for hip fracture. *Aging Clin. Exp. Res.* **2023**, *35*, 1081–1085. [CrossRef]
26. Bohl, D.D.; Shen, M.R.; Hannon, C.P.; Fillingham, Y.A.; Darrith, B.; Della Valle, C.J. Serum albumin predicts survival and postoperative course following surgery for geriatric hip fracture. *J. Bone Jt. Surg. Am.* **2017**, *99*, 2110–2118. [CrossRef] [PubMed]
27. Kieffer, W.K.; Rennie, C.S.; Gandhe, A.J. Preoperative albumin as a predictor of one-year mortality in patients with fractured neck of femur. *Ann. R. Coll. Surg. Engl.* **2013**, *95*, 26–28. [CrossRef] [PubMed]
28. Soliman, S.S.; Jordan, G.B.; Bilaniuk, J.W.; Benfante, A.; Kong, K.; Rolandelli, R.H.; Curran, T.; Nemeth, Z.H. The impact of BMI on morbidity and mortality after femoral fractures. *Eur. J. Trauma Emerg. Surg.* **2022**, *48*, 2441–2447. [CrossRef]
29. Li, J.; Li, D.; Wang, X.; Zhang, L. The impact of body mass index on mortality rates of hip fracture patients: A systematic review and meta-analysis. *Osteoporos. Int.* **2022**, *33*, 1859–1869. [CrossRef]
30. Kregel, H.R.; Murphy, P.B.; Attia, M.; Meyer, D.E.; Morris, R.S.; Onyema, E.C.; Adams, S.D.; Wade, C.E.; Harvin, J.A.; Kao, L.S.; et al. The Geriatric Nutritional Risk Index as a predictor of complications in geriatric trauma patients. *J. Trauma Acute Care Surg.* **2022**, *93*, 195–199. [CrossRef]
31. Zheng, H.; Echave, P.; Mehta, N.; Myrskylä, M. Life-long body mass index trajectories and mortality in two generations. *Ann. Epidemiol.* **2021**, *56*, 18–25. [CrossRef]
32. Aune, D.; Sen, A.; Prasad, M.; Norat, T.; Janszky, I.; Tonstad, S.; Romundstad, P.; Vatten, L.J. BMI and all cause mortality: Systematic review and non-linear dose-response meta-analysis of 230 cohort studies with 3.74 million deaths among 30.3 million participants. *BMJ* **2016**, *4*, 353. [CrossRef]
33. Lv, Y.; Zhang, Y.; Li, X.; Gao, X.; Ren, Y.; Deng, L.; Xu, L.; Zhou, J.; Wu, B.; Wei, Y. Body mass index, waist circumference, and mortality in subjects older than 80 years: A Mendelian randomization study. *Eur. Heart J.* **2024**, *45*, 2145–2154. [CrossRef] [PubMed]
34. Simunovic, N.; Devereaux, P.J.; Sprague, S.; Guyatt, G.H.; Schemitsch, E.; Debeer, J.; Bhandari, M. Effect of early surgery after hip fracture on mortality and complications: A systematic review and meta-analysis. *CMAJ* **2010**, *182*, 1609–1616. [CrossRef]
35. Klestil, T.; Röder, C.; Stotter, C.; Winkler, B.; Nehrer, S.; Lutz, M.; Klerings, I.; Wagner, G.; Gartlehner, G.; Nussbaumer-Streit, B. Impact of timing of surgery in elderly hip fracture patients: A systematic review and meta-analysis. *Sci. Rep.* **2018**, *8*, 13933. [CrossRef]
36. Hamdan, M.; Haddad, B.I.; Almohtasib, J.; Eid, M.; Al-Din, T.J.; Rayyan, H.A.; Altantawi, A.M.; Akaheal, A.S.; Alshrouf, M.A. Postoperative pneumonia after femoral fracture surgery: An in-depth retrospective analysis. *BMC Musculoskelet. Disord.* **2024**, *25*, 413. [CrossRef]
37. Han, S.B.; Kim, S.B.; Shin, K.H. Risk factors for postoperative pneumonia in patients undergoing hip fracture surgery: A systematic review and meta-analysis. *BMC Musculoskelet. Disord.* **2022**, *23*, 553. [CrossRef] [PubMed]
38. Ergin, Ö.N.; Bayram, S.; Anarat, F.B.; Yağcı, T.F.; Balcı, H.İ. Prognostic factors affecting survival of patients with intertrochanteric femoral fractures over 90 years treated with proximal femoral nailing. *Eur. J. Trauma Emerg. Surg.* **2020**, *46*, 663–669. [CrossRef] [PubMed]
39. Oliveira, C.E.N.; Feitosa, A.C.C.; Falótico, G.G.; Ferreira, G.F.; Durigon, T.S.; Arliani, G.G. Mortality in patients > 90 years old with proximal femoral fractures subjected to surgery. *Acta Ortop. Bras.* **2022**, *30*, e255534. [CrossRef]
40. Weinberg, L.; Ou Yang, B.; Cosic, L.; Klink, S.; Le, P.; Li, J.K.; Koshy, A.N.; Jones, D.; Bellomo, R.; Tan, C.O. Factors influencing early and long-term survival following hip fracture among nonagenarians. *J. Orthop. Surg. Res.* **2021**, *16*, 653. [CrossRef]
41. Ogawa, T.; Schermann, H.; Kobayashi, H.; Fushimi, K.; Okawa, A.; Jinno, T. Age and clinical outcomes after hip fracture surgery: Do octogenarian, nonagenarian and centenarian classifications matter? *Age Ageing* **2021**, *50*, 1952–1960. [CrossRef]
42. Ceolin, C.; Bano, G.; Biz, C.; Dianin, M.; Bedogni, M.; Guarnaccia, A.; Berizzi, A.; Ruggieri, P.; Coin, A.; Sergi, G. Functional autonomy and 12-month mortality in older adults with proximal femoral fractures in an orthogeriatric setting: Risk factors and gender differences. *Aging Clin. Exp. Res.* **2023**, *35*, 1063–1071. [CrossRef]
43. van Leendert, J.A.A.; Linkens, A.E.M.J.H.; Poeze, M.; Pijpers, E.; Magdelijns, F.; Ten Broeke, R.H.M.; Spaetgens, B. Mortality in hip fracture patients after implementation of a nurse practitioner-led orthogeriatric care program: Results of a 1-year follow-up. *Age Ageing* **2021**, *50*, 1744–1750. [CrossRef] [PubMed]
44. Spaetgens, B.; Brouns, S.H.A.; Linkens, A.E.M.J.H.; Poeze, M.; Ten Broeke, R.H.M.; Brüggemann, R.A.G.; Sipers, W.; Henry, R.M.A.; Hanssen, N.M.J. Associations between presence of diabetes, mortality and fracture type in individuals with a hip fracture. *Diabetes Res. Clin. Pract.* **2022**, *192*, 110084. [CrossRef] [PubMed]
45. Yan, B.W.; Arias, E.; Geller, A.C.; Miller, D.R.; Kochanek, K.D.; Koh, H.K. Widening gender gap in life expectancy in the US, 2010-2021. *JAMA Intern. Med.* **2024**, *184*, 108–110. [CrossRef]
46. Berry, S.D.; Rothbaum, R.R.; Kiel, D.P.; Lee, Y.; Mitchell, S.L. Association of clinical outcomes with surgical repair of hip fracture vs non-surgical management in nursing home residents with advanced dementia. *JAMA Intern. Med.* **2018**, *178*, 774–780. [CrossRef] [PubMed]

47. Liu, Y.; Zhang, C.W.; Zhao, X.D. Long-term survival of femoral neck fracture patients aged over ninety years: Arthroplast compared with nonoperative treatment. *BMC Musculoskelet. Disord.* **2020**, *21*, 217. [CrossRef]
48. Viganò, M.; Pennestrì, F.; Listorti, E.; Banfi, G. Proximal hip fractures in 71,920 elderly patients: Incidence, epidemiology, mortalit and costs from a retrospective observational study. *BMC Public Health* **2023**, *23*, 1963. [CrossRef]

Journal of Clinical Medicine

MDPI

Article

Trends and Risk Factors for the Hospitalization of Older Adults Presenting to Emergency Departments After a Bed-Related Fall: A National Database Analysis

Andy Tom [1], Sergio M. Navarro [1,2], Grant M. Spears [3], Adam Schluttenhofer [1], Michelle Junker [1], John Zietlow [1], Roderick Davis [1], Allyson K. Palmer [4], Nathan K. LeBrasseur [5], Fernanda Bellolio [6] and Myung S. Park [1,*]

1 Department of Surgery, Division of Trauma, Critical Care and General Surgery, Mayo Clinic, Rochester, MN 55905, USA; tom.andy@mayo.edu (A.T.); navarro.sergio@mayo.edu (S.M.N.); schluttenhofer.adam@mayo.edu (A.S.); junker.michelle@mayo.edu (M.J.); zietlow.john@mayo.edu (J.Z.); davis.roderick@mayo.edu (R.D.)
2 Department of Surgery, University of Minnesota, Minneapolis, MN 55455, USA
3 Department of Quantitative Health Sciences, Mayo Clinic, Rochester, MN 55905, USA; spears.grant@mayo.edu
4 Department of Medicine, Division of Hospital Internal Medicine, Mayo Clinic, Rochester, MN 55905, USA; palmer.allyson@mayo.edu
5 Department of Physical Medicine and Rehabilitation, Mayo Clinic, Rochester, MN 55905, USA; lebrasseur.nathan@mayo.edu
6 Department of Emergency Medicine, Mayo Clinic, Rochester, MN 55905, USA; bellolio.fernanda@mayo.edu
* Correspondence: park.myung@mayo.edu; Tel.: +1-(507)-255-6960; Fax: +1-(507)-255-9872

Abstract: Background/objectives: Falls are a leading cause of traumatic injury and hospitalization for adults over the age of 65. While common, bed-related falls are relatively understudied when compared to ambulatory falls. The aim of this study is to characterize the risk factors for the hospitalization of older adults presenting to U.S. emergency departments (EDs) after a fall from bed. **Methods**: This was a cross-sectional study using publicly available data from the U.S. Consumer Product Safety Commission's National Electronic Injury Surveillance System (NEISS) from 2014 to 2023, including all adults over the age of 65 presenting to the NEISS's participating EDs with bed-related fall injuries. We identified fall injuries using a keyword search of the NEISS narratives and determined how the fall occurred by manually reviewing a randomized 3% sample of the narratives. We summarized demographics and injury patterns with descriptive statistics. We constructed a multivariable logistic regression model to identify risk factors for hospitalization and used Poisson regression to assess temporal trends in fall incidence and hospital admissions. **Results**: An estimated average of 320,751 bed-related fall injuries presented to EDs annually from 2014 to 2023. ED visits increased by 2.85% per year, while hospital admissions rose by 5.67% per year ($p < 0.001$). The most common injury patterns were superficial injuries (contusions, abrasions, lacerations, avulsions, and punctures) (28.6%), fractures (21.7%), and internal injuries (including concussions) (21.6%). Most of the falls occurred while transitioning into or out of bed (34.4%) or falling out of bed (56.8%). Hospitalization was required in 34.1% of cases and was associated with male sex, medication use at time of injury, and fracture injuries. **Conclusions**: Bed-related falls and associated hospitalizations are increasing among older adults. ED providers should understand risk factors for hospitalization in these common injuries such as male sex, medication use at time of injury, and high-risk injury patterns. Additionally, prevention efforts should focus on helping older adults remain safely in bed and then assisting with transitions into or out of bed.

Keywords: older adult; bed-related falls; injury pattern; emergency department; hospitalization

1. Introduction

Falls are the leading cause of injury-related morbidity and mortality in the U.S. for people over the age of 65 [1]. Older adults [defined as adults over the age of 65 are particularly susceptible to serious injury from low-energy falls due to age-related loss of bone mass and bone microstructure, reduced muscle mass, and balance impairment from other comorbidities such as diabetes [2–4]. Increased fall risk is also associated with an increased risk of 30-day mortality after an emergency department (ED) visit for any reason [5]. After falling, many older adults experience lasting impairment from loss of motor capacity, poor gait performance, and depression [6]. As the U.S. population ages, it is increasingly important to understand risk factors associated with falls in this patient population.

Fall injuries are also a significant burden on the finances of individual patients and society as a whole. In 2020, healthcare expenditures for fall injuries in older adults were estimated to exceed USD 80 billion, with the majority being paid by public insurers [7]. Additionally, the median cost to individuals experiencing a fall was USD 26,143, which could be a devastating blow to an already financially vulnerable demographic [8]. There are also additional costs associated with arranging long-term care or transport to follow-up appointments, as well as taking time from work for recovery.

An estimated 3 million falls presented to U.S. EDs in 2015 [9]. Many of these falls are related to consumer products that act as tripping hazards such as stairs, rugs, bathtubs, and toilets [10,11]. While some consumer product-related falls are well characterized in older adults [10–12], traumatic injuries secondary to falling from a bed are less well-studied. Bed-related falls have primarily been examined in a hospital or assisted living setting [13–15], but it is important to understand the number of these injuries that occur nationwide in the community setting. Additionally, traumatic falls from a bed may also present with injury patterns different from ambulatory falls that could guide evaluation in the ED. Lastly, it is important to understand how these injuries occur in the community setting to develop effective risk mitigation strategies.

In this study, we examined the injury patterns and demographic characteristics of older adults who presented to U.S. emergency departments following a bed-related fall from 2014 to 2023. To understand how these injuries occur and what factors lead to hospital admission, we manually reviewed a subset of narratives included in the NEISS data that provide a short description of the events preceding each injury. Additionally, we analyzed factors associated with an increased risk of hospitalization in these patients such as injury pattern, age, medication or alcohol use, and sex [16–18].

2. Materials and Methods

This was a cross-sectional descriptive study using publicly available online data from the U.S. Consumer Product Safety Commission's National Electronic Injury Surveillance System (NEISS). The NEISS collects data on consumer product-related injuries from 100 EDs across the United States selected as a probability sample of all 5000+ U.S. hospitals. When patients with these injuries present to the ED, they are included in the NEISS database [19]. To generate national estimates, the NEISS assigns a weight to each case based on the hospital's annual number of ED visits and geographic location [20].

At NEISS-participating hospitals, a professional coordinator collects standardized data including patient demographics (age and sex), diagnosis, body part injured, patient disposition, location where the injury occurred, and a brief narrative describing the incident that led to the injury. Additionally, the NEISS coordinator assigns each case a consumer product code that specifies a product associated with the injury [19]. Data from the NEISS has been used previously to characterize consumer product-related injury trends [10–12]. We adhere to the Strengthening the Reporting of Observational Studies in Epidemiology (STROBE) guidelines for reporting observational studies [21].

This study utilized publicly available data and was determined not to require Institutional Review Board (IRB) review or approval. The data used in this research is accessible to the public without any restrictions, ensuring that no identifiable information about individuals is included.

We queried the NEISS for product codes in the "Beds, mattresses, and pillows" category and included all patients ≥65 years old from 2014 to 2023 that presented after an injury to a NEISS-participating ED. We filtered for fall injuries by searching the narrative for keywords related to falls (i.e., fall, fell, etc.) and categorized bed-related injuries as "fall" or "non-fall." We used the NEISS sampling weights to obtain national estimates and trends of bed-related fall injuries over the study period, as well as demographic and injury-related characteristics of these patients [20].

We randomly selected a sample of 3% (n = 2112) of the bed-related fall cohort for manual review. The 3% was based on the necessary sample size for estimating event proportions, based on a population of 70,391 cases, with a 2% margin of error and 95% confidence interval [22,23]. In the bed-related fall cohort, we reviewed the narrative for each injury and sorted injuries into one of the following categories:

1. Falling out of bed—incidents where the patient fell out of bed while they were already safely in bed.
2. Transitioning—falling during a transition into or out of bed.
3. During activity out of bed—falls that occurred when the patient was out of bed performing some activity (i.e., making the bed, vacuuming around the bed and tripped on bedframe, etc.).
4. Found down/other—patient was found down by someone else and unable to report mechanism or fall was due to a unique mechanism (i.e., trying to exercise sitting on edge of bed and fell).
5. Incorrectly labeled fall—injuries that were incorrectly identified as falls (n = 59, 2.8%). These were excluded from subsequent analyses.

We also reviewed the "body part" and "diagnosis" codes designated by the NEISS and combined them into the following "injury pattern" categories using a modified Barell matrix [24]: lower trunk fractures/dislocations, upper trunk fractures/dislocations, lower extremity fractures/dislocations, upper extremity fractures/dislocations, head/face/neck fractures, internal injuries (including hematomas and concussions), pain/weakness, contusions/abrasions/lacerations/avulsions/punctures, sprains/strains, and other/unspecified.

We report descriptive statistics as median (IQR) or frequency (%) and display the data three ways for comparison—as an unweighted summary of the full NEISS bed-related falls cohort, as weighted estimates for the full U.S. population based on the full cohort and each patient's associated NEISS sample weight, and finally as an unweighted summary of the manually reviewed 3% subsample (after removing the incorrectly included non-fall injuries). To conduct a trend analysis of falls over time, within the full bed-related falls cohort, we fitted Poisson regression models to assess changes in the number of fall-related ED visits and resulting hospitalizations over time, with year as the independent variable. We adjusted these counts by dividing by the total number of ED visits per year among geriatric patients to account for annual fluctuations in total ED visits. We assessed the goodness of fit of the Poisson regression models with McFadden's pseudo-R-squared.

Using the subsample of manually reviewed cases, we analyzed risk factors for hospitalization after presentation to the ED with logistic regression. We analyzed demographic and injury-related characteristics in a simple regression model and considered variables with a p-value less than 0.10 for inclusion in a multivariable regression model. Because data was only available from 2018 to 2023 regarding the contribution of medications to the fall incidents, we constructed a secondary multivariable model including this variable on data from that time frame. All statistical analyses were completed using R (version 4.3.0; R Core Team, 2024).

3. Results

Table 1 includes the demographics and injury characteristics of the cohort. From 2014 to 2023, a total of 70,391 patients with bed-related falls presented to NEISS-participating EDs, with an average of 7039 bed-related falls per year. This translated to a mean national estimate of 320,751 (SD 58,218) bed-related injuries per year. Over the study period, after accounting for sampling weights, the estimated median patient age was 81 (IQR 73–88), with 36.3% men and 63.7% women. An estimated 64.2% of injuries were treated and released from the ED, 35.1% required hospitalization, observation, or subsequent transfer, 0.5% left without being seen, and 0.1% resulted in mortality. Superficial injuries (contusions/abrasions/lacerations/avulsions) were the most common injury pattern with a frequency of 28.6%, fracture and dislocations accounted for 21.7%, and internal injuries (including concussions) accounted for 21.6%.

Table 1. Demographic and injury characteristics.

		NEISS Bed-Related Falls Raw Total (n = 70,391)	Weighted U.S. Estimate (n = 3,207,432)	Manually Reviewed Sample Raw Total (n = 2053)
Age	Median (IQR)	81 (73, 88)	81 (73, 88)	81 (74-88)
Sex	Male	25,677 (36.5%)	1,163,366 (36.3%)	735 (35.8%)
	Female	44,713 (63.5%)	2,044,066 (63.7%)	1318 (64.2%)
	Intersex	1 (0.0%)	80 (0.0%)	-
Hospitalized	Yes	23,975 (34.1%)	1,054,858 (32.9%)	699 (34.0%)
	No	46,416 (65.9%)	2,152,655 (67.1%)	1354 (66.0%)
Disposition	Treated and Released	44,203 (62.8%)	2,060,395 (64.2%)	1284 (62.5%)
	Treated and Transferred	1072 (1.5%)	67,590 (2.1%)	28 (1.4%)
	Treated and Hospitalized	22,903 (32.5%)	987,268 (30.8%)	671 (32.7%)
	Held for Observation	1750 (2.5%)	72,406 (2.3%)	55 (2.7%)
	Left without Being Seen	368 (0.5%)	16,096 (0.5%)	10 (0.5%)
	Fatality	95 (0.1%)	3757 (0.1%)	5 (0.2%)
Alcohol [1]	Yes	440 (1.1%)	19,967 (1.1%)	13 (1.1%)
	No	39,932 (98.9%)	1,805,797 (98.9%)	1177 (98.9%)
Drug/Medication Caused [1]	Yes	1736 (4.3%)	70,302 (3.9%)	55 (4.6%)
	No	38,636 (95.7%)	1,755,462 (96.1%)	1135 (95.4%)
Injury Pattern	Lower Trunk Fracture/Dislocation	5965 (8.5%)	271,325 (8.5%)	170 (8.3%)
	Lower Extremity Fracture/Dislocation	2607 (3.7%)	119,724 (3.7%)	79 (3.8%)
	Other/Unspecified	7987 (11.3%)	358,754 (11.2%)	221 (10.8%)
	Upper Trunk Fracture/Dislocation	2282 (3.2%)	104,235 (3.2%)	79 (3.8%)

Table 1. *Cont.*

		NEISS Bed-Related Falls Raw Total (n = 70,391)	Weighted U.S. Estimate (n = 3,207,432)	Manually Reviewed Sample Raw Total (n = 2053)
	Head/Face/Neck Fracture/Dislocation	1256 (1.8%)	53,914 (1.7%)	32 (1.6%)
	Internal Injury (incl. Concussions)	16,310 (23.2%)	692,911 (21.6%)	513 (25.0%)
	Pain/Weakness	9574 (13.6%)	416,635 (13.0%)	262 (12.8%)
	Upper Extremity Fracture/Dislocation	3081 (4.4%)	145,776 (4.5%)	106 (5.2%)
	Superficial (Contusions/Abrasions/Lacerations/Avulsions)	18,641 (26.5%)	918,711 (28.6%)	521 (25.4%)
	Sprains/Strains	2688 (3.8%)	125,528 (3.9%)	70 (3.4%)
Injury Mechanism [2]	In Bed (Fell Out/Rolled)	-	-	1167 (56.8%)
	Transitioning	-	-	707 (34.4%)
	Out of Bed (Walking/Activity)	-	-	122 (5.9%)
	Other/Unclear	-	-	57 (2.8%)

[1] Data only available for fall injuries from 2018–2023. [2] Data only available for manually reviewed sample.

The number of ED visits for bed-related falls (as a fraction of total ED visits) increased by an average of 2.85% each year over the study period (95% CI 2.64–3.06%, $p < 0.001$), and hospital admissions due to falls (also as a fraction of total ED visits) increased by an average of 5.67% each year (95% CI 5.29–6.05, $p < 0.001$) (Figures 1 and 2).

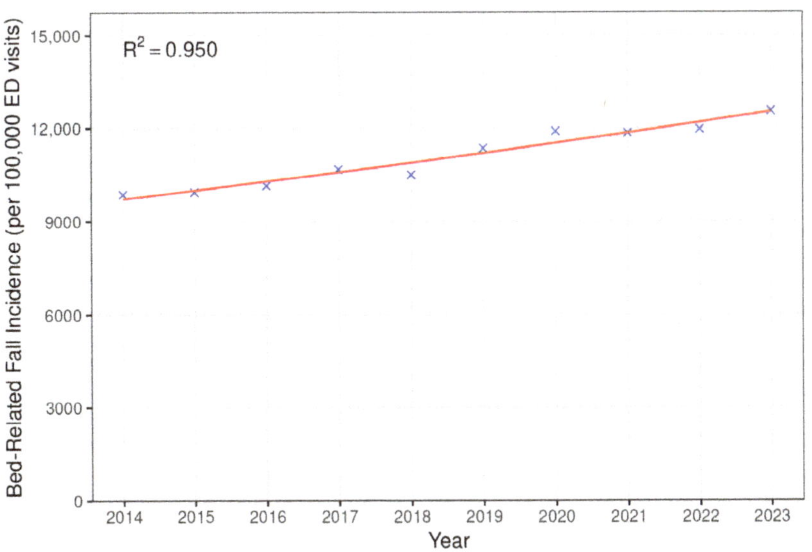

Figure 1. Trends in national estimated ED visits for bed-related falls.

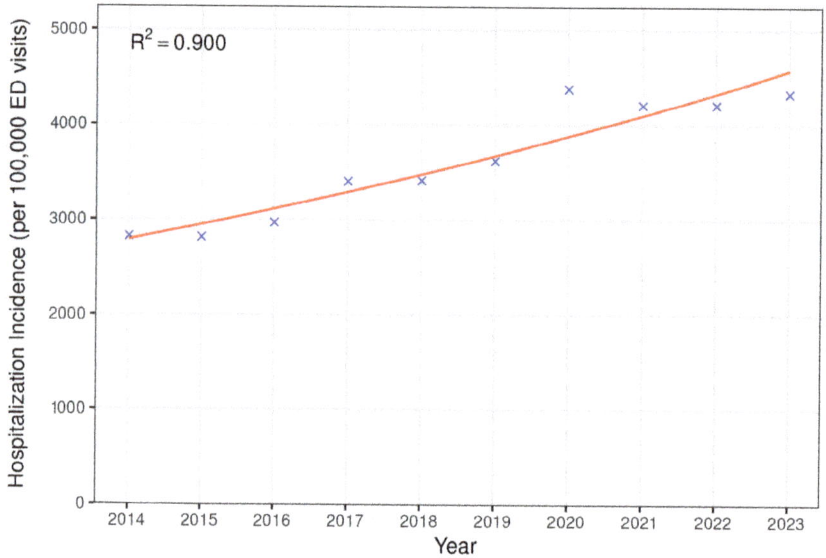

Figure 2. Trends in hospitalization for bed-related falls.

In the selected subsample, which was manually reviewed and categorized by mechanism of injury, a total of 56.8% of falls occurred while in bed, 34.4% occurred during a transition into or out of bed, 5.9% occurred during an activity out of the bed, and in 2.8%, the mechanism and involvement of the bed in the injury was unique or unable to be determined.

Results of the univariate logistic analyses are presented in Table 2. Men were more likely to require hospitalization and have injuries associated with medication use. Hospitalization rates were also significantly associated with injury patterns. Injury mechanism was borderline significant ($p = 0.088$), with hospitalization occurring most frequently in patients with injuries while transitioning in and out of bed. Age and alcohol use at time of injury did not meet our threshold for significance.

Based on the selection criteria ($p < 0.10$), sex, injury pattern, and injury mechanism were included in the multivariable model on all patients from 2014 to 2023 (Table 3). Men remained more likely to be admitted to the hospital compared to women (OR = 1.55, 95% CI: 1.26–1.91, $p < 0.001$). Among injury patterns, lower trunk fractures (OR = 10.04, 95% CI: 6.41–16.06 vs. patients diagnosed with pain/weakness) and lower extremity fractures (OR = 4.59, 95% CI: 2.71–7.88) were associated with the highest odds of hospitalization. Other significant injury patterns associated with increased hospitalization included other/unspecified injuries (OR = 2.52, 95% CI: 1.72–3.70), upper trunk fractures (OR = 2.23, 95% CI: 1.31–3.77), and head/neck/face fractures or dislocations (OR = 2.17, 95% CI: 1.01–4.61). Conversely, patients with superficial injuries (OR = 0.56, 95% CI: 0.39–0.80) and patients with sprains or strains (OR = 0.30, 95% CI: 0.12–0.66) were significantly less likely to be hospitalized compared to patients presenting with pain or weakness. Injury mechanism was not significantly associated with hospitalization in the multivariable model ($p = 0.59$). A secondary multivariable model (Table 4) was run on patients injured from 2018 to 2023, as data collected during this timeframe included information about whether medication/drug use contributed to each bed-related fall. In this model, falls caused by drug or medication use were associated with a higher likelihood of hospitalization (OR = 2.13, 95% CI: 1.20–3.80, $p = 0.010$).

Table 2. Univariate analysis identifying predictors of hospitalization.

Variable	Level	N Total	N Hospitalized	% Hospitalized	OR	95% CI	p-Value
Age	Per 10 years	-	-	-	1.07	0.97, 1.18	0.19
Sex	Male	735	285	38.8%	1.38	1.15, 1.67	**<0.001**
	Female	1318	414	31.4%	1.00	Ref	
Alcohol [1]	Yes	13	7	53.8%	2.00	0.66, 6.24	0.22
	No	1177	434	36.9%	1.00	Ref	
Drug/Medication Caused [1]	Yes	55	29	52.7%	1.96	1.14, 3.39	**0.015**
	No	1135	412	36.3%	1.00	Ref	
Injury Pattern							**<0.001**
	Lower Trunk Fracture	170	133	78.2%	9.86	6.31, 15.72	
	Lower Extremity Fracture	79	48	60.8%	4.25	2.52, 7.26	
	Other/Unspecified	221	123	55.7%	2.62	1.80, 3.85	
	Upper Trunk Fracture	79	35	44.3%	2.18	1.29, 3.68	
	Head/Neck/Face Fracture/Dislocation	32	14	43.8%	2.13	0.99, 4.51	
	Internal Injury (incl. Concussions)	513	167	32.6%	1.32	0.96, 1.85	
	Pain/Weakness	262	70	26.7%	1.00	Ref	
	Upper Extremity Fracture	106	27	25.5%	0.94	0.55, 1.56	
	Superficial (Contusions/Abrasions/ Lacerations/Avulsions)	521	90	17.3%	0.57	0.40, 0.82	
	Sprains/Strains	70	7	10.0%	0.31	0.12, 0.66	
Injury Mechanism							**0.088**
	In Bed (Fell Out/Rolled)	1167	384	32.9%	1.22	0.82, 1.86	
	Transitioning	707	264	37.3%	1.48	0.98, 2.28	
	Out of Bed (Walking/Activity)	124	35	28.2%	1.00	Ref	
	Other/Unclear	57	16	28.1%	0.97	0.47, 1.93	

[1] Data only available for fall injuries from 2018–2023. **Bold** used to denote p-values that are significant (<0.05).

Table 3. Multivariable logistic regression analysis of risk factors for hospital admission following falls using covariates with $p < 0.10$ in univariate analysis.

Predictor	Level	OR	95% CI	p-Value
Sex	Male	1.55	1.26, 1.91	**<0.001**
	Female	1.00	Ref	
Injury Pattern				**<0.001**
	Lower Trunk Fracture	10.04	6.41, 16.06	
	Lower Extremity Fracture	4.59	2.71, 7.88	
	Other/Unspecified	2.52	1.72, 3.70	
	Upper Trunk Fracture	2.23	1.31, 3.77	
	Head/Neck/Face Fracture/Dislocation	2.17	1.01, 4.61	
	Internal Injury (incl. Concussions)	1.30	0.94, 1.83	
	Pain/Weakness	1.00	Ref	
	Upper Extremity Fracture	0.99	0.58, 1.64	
	Superficial (Contusions/Abrasions/ Lacerations/Avulsions)	0.56	0.39, 0.80	
	Sprains/Strains	0.30	0.12, 0.66	

Table 3. *Cont.*

Predictor	Level	OR	95% CI	p-Value
Injury Mechanism				0.59
	In Bed (Fell Out/Rolled)	1.27	0.81, 2.02	
	Transitioning	1.37	0.86, 2.20	
	Out of Bed (Walking/Activity)	1.00	Ref	
	Other/Unclear	1.16	0.54, 2.43	

Bold used to denote *p*-values that are significant (<0.05).

Table 4. Multivariable logistic regression analysis of risk factors for hospital admission following falls using covariates $p < 0.10$ in univariate analysis with only patients injured from 2018 to 2023 when medication data was available.

Predictor	Level	OR	95% CI	p-Value
Sex	Male	1.44	1.11, 1.88	**0.007**
	Female	1.00	Ref	
Drugs/Medications	Yes	2.13	1.20, 3.80	**0.010**
	No	1.00	Ref	
Injury Pattern				**<0.001**
	Lower Trunk Fracture	7.98	4.55, 14.43	
	Lower Extremity Fracture	3.35	1.74, 6.58	
	Other/Unspecified	2.05	1.29, 3.27	
	Upper Trunk Fracture	1.54	0.77, 3.06	
	Head/Neck/Face Fracture/Dislocation	1.43	0.53, 3.71	
	Internal Injury (incl. Concussions)	0.90	0.59, 1.37	
	Pain/Weakness	1.00	Ref	
	Upper Extremity Fracture	0.76	0.35, 1.55	
	Superficial (Contusions/Abrasions/ Lacerations/Avulsions)	0.57	0.36, 0.89	
	Sprains/Strains	0.15	0.02, 0.52	
Injury Mechanism				0.74
	In Bed (Fell Out/Rolled)	1.37	0.77, 2.53	
	Transitioning	1.39	0.77, 2.59	
	Out of Bed (Walking/Activity)	1.00	Ref	
	Other/Unclear	1.22	0.48, 3.03	

Bold used to denote *p*-values that are significant (<0.05).

4. Discussion

Our study investigated fall injuries involving a bed in older adults using a national database. Bed-related falls represent approximately 10% of the estimated 3 million falls in adults over 65 that presented to the ED in 2015 [9]. We found that bed-related fall injuries and hospitalizations have increased at a rate of 2.85% annually compared to a 3% annual increase for all consumer product-related injuries in this age group [19]. This increase mirrors a broader trend of rising fall injuries and mortality from falls [25], likely driven by increasing multimorbidity in the U.S. [26].

When examining bed-related injuries, we found that 12.8% of cases sub-sampled included ED presentations due to pain and general weakness, a category that is not part of the original NEISS coding. These cases do not fit well into a traditional injury classification scheme; however, older patients with generalized weakness are more likely to sustain an injury [27], and older patients who present to the ED with non-specific complaints have a high risk of hospitalization and 30-day mortality [28,29]. The 12.8% of patients presenting with pain/weakness in our cohort highlights the importance of a comprehensive assessment of older adults presenting to the ED after a fall and incorporating gait evaluation prior to dismissal to ensure safety [30]. Furthermore, falls in older adults represent a sentinel event and a marker for deterioration in their health [31]. Reducing fall-related injury begins with prehospital evaluations and "lift assist" calls and continues through risk assessments, screenings, and interventions that occur during and after emergency department visits [31].

A total of 36.7% of bed-related falls identified required subsequent hospitalization or transfer. Previous studies have shown that risk factors for hospitalization after a fall include diagnoses of Parkinson's dementia and urinary tract infection, as well as low functional status and physical activity [32]. Our study found that certain injury patterns, medication use, and sex were risk factors for hospitalization. While women were more likely to present to the ED, men were more likely to require hospitalization. Men were also more likely to fall once hospitalized and are more likely to experience fall-related mortality, indicating that men may present to the hospital with more severe injuries relative to their health status than women [1,33]. Interestingly, age was not an independent risk factor for hospitalization in our cohort, indicating that other factors such as injury pattern and medication use are more important drivers of hospitalization. Other risk factors for hospitalization included fracture or dislocation of any type. These injuries were some of the most common injuries in our cohort, highlighting the need for a thorough musculoskeletal evaluation, including an evaluation for rib fractures after a bed-related fall. Injuries associated with prescription medications were also more likely to require hospitalization. The association between medications and hospitalization should prompt a medication review in older adults presenting to the ED after a fall. While internal injuries, most of which were head injuries, were not associated with an increased risk of admission in our cohort, these injuries have been associated with an increased risk of return to the ED within 90 days and should be followed up closely [34].

Polypharmacy, the use of high-risk medications like benzodiazepines or opioids [35,36], high comorbidity burden, visual and hearing impairments, orthostatic hypotension, home hazards, balance and gait abnormalities, sarcopenia, alcohol use disorder, and frailty are known risk factors for falls [37,38]. Identifying and addressing modifiable risk factors such as poor visual acuity, high-risk medication use, and gait abnormalities during ED and routine clinic visits prevent recurrent falls and promote safer mobility [39]. Measures of function collected at the index ED visit, such as the Timed Up and Go, are helpful in predicting clinical outcomes [40]. The American Geriatrics Society and the Geriatric Emergency Care Applied Research Network (GEAR) emphasize comprehensive fall risk assessments, including medication reviews and environmental evaluations, as part of their guidelines for geriatric emergency care [41].

The mechanisms we identified through our narrative analysis provide valuable insight for prevention efforts. Falling out of bed while already in bed accounted for 56.8% of injuries, while falls during a transition into or out of bed represented 34.4% of injuries. Interestingly, falls occurring while the patient was out of bed, such as tripping over the bed frame or falling while making the bed, were less frequent at 5.9% but still warrant attention as part of a comprehensive fall prevention strategy. Previous studies have demonstrated that falls are associated with decline in function in more than one third of the patients [37]. Our findings suggest that while fall mechanism was a significant risk factor for hospitalization in the univariate analysis, injury pattern, especially fractures, was the most important driver of hospitalization risk. This may be because certain fall mechanisms such as transitioning could lead to more severe injuries; thus, the mechanism and injury pattern may be dependent on one another.

While physical measures such as bed rails, compliant flooring, and low-level beds have not been shown to reduce bed-related fall injuries in hospital and long-term care settings, these interventions have not been evaluated in older adults living independently [13–15]. Exercise plans have been shown to reduce the risk of falling and risk of serious injury after a fall and could help reduce the risk of falling while transitioning into or out of bed [42]. Additionally, multifactorial plans that include an assessment (timed up and go test, gait speed test, Berg balance scale, etc.), a medication review, and one or more additional interventions based on individual risk factors have been shown to be effective at reducing falls, in general, but were not specifically targeted toward bed-related falls [42]. Our research suggests that interventions focused on helping older adults remain safely in their beds during rest and move in and out of their beds could have the greatest impact on reducing bed-related falls.

Our research had several limitations. The NEISS collects data from a nationally representative sample of EDs but does not include a validated injury severity score and does not account for non-emergent injuries treated at community clinics. As a result, the database likely underestimates the total incidence of bed-related fall injuries. Furthermore, the NEISS captures presentations to EDs from the community but may not capture bed-related fall injuries occurring during hospitalization. Additionally, while the narratives provide a useful source of supplementary information, they are not standardized and can vary in their content. The lack of standardized reporting in the narratives could potentially introduce non-differential misclassification bias, although the analysis of the narratives has been validated in case–control studies [43]. The coding structure of the NEISS can also lack specificity on the diagnoses [44], data quality and completeness rely on documentation available from the medical records, and the NEISS only includes drug and alcohol data starting in 2018. Lastly, the NEISS only records information during the initial presentation to the ED, precluding any long-term follow-up or analysis.

While our study provides a basic understanding of the epidemiology and risk factors for hospitalization for bed-related falls, more research is needed to find interventions effective at preventing these injuries. The current study highlights the need for targeted efforts to reduce fall-related injuries in the bed environment [42]. Additionally, ongoing research is primarily focused on preventing these injuries in hospital wards or assisted living settings [13–15]. Future research is needed on evaluating interventions for older adults who are at risk of falling but live independently in the community.

5. Conclusions

The incidence of bed-related falls and significant injuries requiring hospitalization has been increasing in the past decade. This trend will most likely continue as the U.S. population ages. Our study provides insight into the trends, mechanisms, and injury patterns of bed-related falls in the geriatric (≥65 years old) population. One third of patients who present to an ED following a bed-related fall will require subsequent hospitalization. Patients with nonspecific complaints such as pain and weakness were much more likely to require hospitalization than patients with superficial injuries, highlighting the need for comprehensive assessment in all patients presenting with falls, including those that have no evident injuries. Fracture injuries—particularly lower trunk and lower extremity fractures—alongside drug/medication use and male sex emerged as the strongest predictors of hospitalization after falls. Understanding these patterns and trends is vital to guiding patient counseling and future preventative efforts.

Author Contributions: Conceptualization, A.T., S.M.N., M.J., J.Z., R.D., M.S.P., F.B., A.K.P. and N.K.L.; methodology, A.T., S.M.N., M.J., J.Z., R.D., M.S.P., F.B., A.K.P. and N.K.L.; validation, A.T., A.S. and G.M.S.; formal analysis, A.T., S.M.N., A.S. and G.M.S.; investigation, A.T., S.M.N., A.S. and G.M.S.; data curation, A.T., A.S. and G.M.S.; writing—original draft preparation, A.T.; funding acquisition, S.M.N. and M.S.P.; writing—review and editing, A.T., S.M.N., A.S., G.M.S., M.J., J.Z., R.D., M.S.P., F.B., A.K.P. and N.K.L.; visualization, A.T., A.S. and G.M.S.; supervision, M.S.P.; project administration, S.M.N. All authors have read and agreed to the published version of the manuscript.

Funding: This project was supported by the Mayo Clinic Robert and Arlene Kogod Center on Aging and R01HL162729-02 (MSP), R38HL150086 Stimulating Access to Research in Residency (SMN), and UL1 TR002377 (MSP) from the National Center for Advancing Translational Sciences.

Institutional Review Board Statement: This study utilized publicly available data, which does not require IRB approval. The data used in this research is accessible to the public without any restrictions, ensuring that no identifiable information about individuals is included.

Informed Consent Statement: Patient consent was waived as the data used in this research is accessible to the public without any restrictions, ensuring that no identifiable information about individuals is included.

Data Availability Statement: The data supporting the conclusions of this article are available from https://www.cpsc.gov/cgibin/NEISSQuery/home.aspx (accessed on 24 October 2024).

Acknowledgments: This article is a revised and expanded version of a paper entitled "Increasing Incidence and Hospitalization of Bed-Related Fall Injuries in Older Adults", which was presented at the American Geriatric Society 2025 Annual Meeting, Chicago, IL, USA, 8–10 May 2025 [45].

Conflicts of Interest: The authors declare no conflicts of interest. The funders had no role in the design of the study; in the collection, analyses, or interpretation of data; in the writing of the manuscript; or in the decision to publish the results.

Abbreviations

The following abbreviations are used in this manuscript:

NEISS	National electronic injury surveillance system
ED	Emergency department
STROBE	Strengthening the Reporting of Observational Studies in Epidemiology
IRB	Institutional Review Board
GEAR	Geriatric Emergency Care Applied Research Network

References

1. Kakara, R.; Bergen, G.; Burns, E.; Stevens, M. Nonfatal and Fatal Falls Among Adults Aged $\geq$ 65 Years—United States, 2020-2021. *MMWR Morb. Mortal. Wkly. Rep.* **2023**, *72*, 938–943. [CrossRef] [PubMed]
2. Reeve, J.; Loveridge, N. The fragile elderly hip: Mechanisms associated with age-related loss of strength and toughness. *Bone* **2014**, *61*, 138–148. [CrossRef] [PubMed]
3. Yamada, M.; Kimura, Y.; Ishiyama, D.; Otobe, Y.; Suzuki, M.; Koyama, S.; Arai, H. Combined effect of lower muscle quality and quantity on incident falls and fall-related fractures in community-dwelling older adults: A 3-year follow-up study. *Bone* **2022**, *162*, 116474. [CrossRef] [PubMed]
4. Wallace, C.; Reiber, G.E.; LeMaster, J.; Smith, D.G.; Sullivan, K.; Hayes, S.; Vath, C. Incidence of falls, risk factors for falls, and fall-related fractures in individuals with diabetes and a prior foot ulcer. *Diabetes Care* **2002**, *25*, 1983–1986. [CrossRef] [PubMed]
5. Hamilton, M.P.; Bellolio, F.; Jeffery, M.M.; Bower, S.M.; Palmer, A.K.; Tung, E.E.; Mullan, A.F.; Carpenter, C.R.; Oliveira, J.E.S.L. Risk of falls is associated with 30-day mortality among older adults in the emergency department. *Am. J. Emerg. Med.* **2024**, *79*, 122–126. [CrossRef] [PubMed]
6. Park, C.; Atique, M.M.U.; Mishra, R.; Najafi, B. Association between Fall History and Gait, Balance, Physical Activity, Depression, Fear of Falling, and Motor Capacity: A 6-Month Follow-Up Study. *Int. J. Environ. Res. Public Health* **2022**, *19*, 10785. [CrossRef] [PubMed]

7. Haddad, Y.K.; Miller, G.F.; Kakara, R.; Florence, C.; Bergen, G.; Burns, E.R.; Atherly, A. Healthcare spending for non-fatal fall among older adults, USA. *Inj. Prev.* **2024**, *30*, 272–276. [CrossRef] [PubMed]
8. Newgard, C.D.; Lin, A.; Caughey, A.B.; Eckstrom, E.; Bulger, E.M.; Staudenmayer, K.; Maughan, B.; Malveau, S.; Griffiths, D McConnell, K.J. The Cost of a Fall Among Older Adults Requiring Emergency Services. *J. Am. Geriatr. Soc.* **2021**, *69*, 389–39 [CrossRef] [PubMed]
9. Moreland, B.L.; Kakara, R.; Haddad, Y.K.; Shakya, I.; Bergen, G. A Descriptive Analysis of Location of Older Adult Falls Tha Resulted in Emergency Department Visits in the United States, 2015. *Am. J. Lifestyle Med.* **2021**, *15*, 590–597. [CrossRef] [PubMed
10. Solaiman, R.H.; Irfanullah, E.; Navarro, S.M.; Keil, E.J.; Onizuka, N.; Tompkins, M.A.; Harmon, J.V., Jr. Rising incidence o stair-related upper extremity fractures among older adults in the United States: A 10-year nationwide analysis. *Osteoporos. In* **2023**, *34*, 1241–1248. [CrossRef] [PubMed]
11. Shields, W.; Omaki, E.; Aassar, M.L.; Blue, T.; Brooks, B.; O'Hara, J.; Perona, R.Y. Structural housing elements associated wit injuries in older adults in the USA. *Inj. Prev.* **2024**, Aug 6:ip-2024-045252. [CrossRef] [PubMed]
12. Orces, C.H. Emergency department visits for fall-related fractures among older adults in the USA: A retrospective cross-sectiona analysis of the National Electronic Injury Surveillance System All Injury Program, 2001–2008. *BMJ Open* **2013**, *3*, e00172 [CrossRef] [PubMed]
13. Capezuti, E.; Maislin, G.; Strumpf, N.; Evans, L.K. Side rail use and bed-related fall outcomes among nursing home resident *J. Am. Geriatr. Soc.* **2002**, *50*, 90–96. [CrossRef] [PubMed]
14. Mackey, D.C.; Lachance, C.C.; Wang, P.T.; Feldman, F.; Laing, A.C.; Leung, P.M.; Hu, X.J.; Robinovitch, S.N. The Flooring fo Injury Prevention (FLIP) Study of compliant flooring for the prevention of fall-related injuries in long-term care: A randomize trial. *PLoS Med.* **2019**, *16*, e1002843. [CrossRef] [PubMed]
15. Haines, T.P.; Bell, R.A.; Varghese, P.N. Pragmatic, cluster randomized trial of a policy to introduce low-low beds to hospital ward for the prevention of falls and fall injuries. *J. Am. Geriatr. Soc.* **2010**, *58*, 435–441. [CrossRef] [PubMed]
16. Zaninotto, P.; Huang, Y.T.; Di Gessa, G.; Abell, J.; Lassale, C.; Steptoe, A. Polypharmacy is a risk factor for hospital admission du to a fall: Evidence from the English Longitudinal Study of Ageing. *BMC Public Health* **2020**, *20*, 1804. [CrossRef] [PubMed]
17. Lo, A.X.; Flood, K.L.; Biese, K.; Platts-Mills, T.F.; Donnelly, J.P.; Carpenter, C.R. Factors Associated With Hospital Admission fo Older Adults Receiving Care in U.S. Emergency Departments. *J. Gerontol. A Biol. Sci. Med. Sci.* **2017**, *72*, 1105–1109. [CrossRef [PubMed]
18. Schroeder, T.J.; Rodgers, G.B. Factors associated with the hospital admission of consumer product-related injuries treated in U.S hospital emergency departments. *Accid. Anal. Prev.* **2013**, *59*, 566–573. [CrossRef] [PubMed]
19. U.S. Consumer Product Safety Commission. National Electronic Injury Surveillance System. Available online: https://www.cpsc gov/Research--Statistics/NEISS-Injury-Data/Neiss-Frequently-Asked-Questions (accessed on 12 November 2024).
20. Schroeder, T.; Ault, K. *The NEISS Sample (Design and Implementation) 1997 to Present*; U.S. Consumer Product Safety Commission Bethesda, MD, USA, 2001.
21. von Elm, E.; Altman, D.G.; Egger, M.; Pocock, S.J.; Gøtzsche, P.C.; Vandenbroucke, J.P. The Strengthening the Reporting of Observational Studies in Epidemiology (STROBE) statement: Guidelines for reporting observational studies. *Ann. Intern. Med* **2007**, *147*, 573–577. [CrossRef] [PubMed]
22. Fox, N.; Hunn, A.; Mathers, N. Sampling and Sample Size Calculation. The NIHR RDS for the East Midlands/Yorkshire & the Humber 2007. Available online: https://www.researchgate.net/profile/Mansour-Abdullah-Alshehri/post/How_to_determine_population_and_sample_size_for_a_survey_research/attachment/5aa18dfc4cde266d58902255/AS:601990316974080@1520537084240/download/Sampling+Sample+Size+Calculation.pdf (accessed on 9 July 2025).
23. Peduzzi, P.; Concato, J.; Kemper, E.; Holford, T.R.; Feinstein, A.R. A simulation study of the number of events per variable in logistic regression analysis. *J. Clin. Epidemiol.* **1996**, *49*, 1373–1379. [CrossRef] [PubMed]
24. Barell, V.; Aharonson-Daniel, L.; Fingerhut, L.A.; Mackenzie, E.J.; Ziv, A.; Boyko, V.; Abargel, A.; Avitzour, M.; Heruti, R. An introduction to the Barell body region by nature of injury diagnosis matrix. *Inj. Prev.* **2002**, *8*, 91–96. [CrossRef] [PubMed]
25. Kendrick, P.; Kelly, Y.O.; Baumann, M.M.; Kahn, E.; Compton, K.; Schmidt, C.; Sylte, D.O.; Li, Z.; La Motte-Kerr, W. Daoud, F.; et al. Mortality due to falls by county, age group, race, and ethnicity in the USA, 2000–2019: A systematic analysis of health disparities. *Lancet Public Health* **2024**, *9*, e539–e550. [CrossRef] [PubMed]
26. Bishop, N.J.; Haas, S.A.; Quiñones, A.R. Cohort Trends in the Burden of Multiple Chronic Conditions Among Aging U.S. Adults *J. Gerontol. B Psychol. Sci. Soc. Sci.* **2022**, *77*, 1867–1879. [CrossRef] [PubMed]
27. Middleton, R.; Poveda, J.L.; Orfila Pernas, F.; Martinez Laguna, D.; Diez Perez, A.; Nogués, X.; Carbonell Abella, C.; Reyes, C. Prieto-Alhambra, D. Mortality, Falls, and Fracture Risk Are Positively Associated With Frailty: A SIDIAP Cohort Study of 890 000 Patients. *J. Gerontol. A Biol. Sci. Med. Sci.* **2022**, *77*, 148–154. [CrossRef] [PubMed]
28. Erwander, K.; Ivarsson, K.; Olsson, M.L.; Agvall, B. Elderly patients with non-specific complaints at the emergency department have a high risk for admission and 30-days mortality. *BMC Geriatr.* **2024**, *24*, 5. [CrossRef] [PubMed]

29. van Dam, C.S.; Peters, M.J.L.; Hoogendijk, E.O.; Nanayakkara, P.W.B.; Muller, M.; Trappenburg, M.C. Older patients with nonspecific complaints at the Emergency Department are at risk of adverse health outcomes. *Eur. J. Intern. Med.* **2023**, *112*, 86–92. [CrossRef] [PubMed]
30. Sanford, A.M.; Morley, J.E.; Berg-Weger, M.; Lundy, J.; Little, M.O.; Leonard, K.; Malmstrom, T.K. High prevalence of geriatric syndromes in older adults. *PLoS ONE* **2020**, *15*, e0233857. [CrossRef] [PubMed]
31. Carpenter, C.R.; Cameron, A.; Ganz, D.A.; Liu, S. Older Adult Falls in Emergency Medicine-A Sentinel Event. *Clin. Geriatr. Med.* **2018**, *34*, 355–367. [CrossRef] [PubMed]
32. Abell, J.G.; Lassale, C.; Batty, G.D.; Zaninotto, P. Risk Factors for Hospital Admission After a Fall: A Prospective Cohort Study of Community-Dwelling Older People. *J. Gerontol. A Biol. Sci. Med. Sci.* **2021**, *76*, 666–674. [CrossRef] [PubMed]
33. Berecki-Gisolf, J.; Rezaei-Darzi, E.; Natora, A.H. Gender differences in the incidence, characteristics and hospital admission outcomes of fall-related injuries in older adults in Victoria, Australia, over 5 years from 2018/19 to 2022/23. *Front. Public Health* **2024**, *12*, 1426726. [CrossRef] [PubMed]
34. Southerland, L.T.; Stephens, J.A.; Robinson, S.; Falk, J.; Phieffer, L.; Rosenthal, J.A.; Caterino, J.M. Head Trauma from Falling Increases Subsequent Emergency Department Visits More Than Other Fall-Related Injuries in Older Adults. *J. Am. Geriatr. Soc.* **2016**, *64*, 870–874. [CrossRef] [PubMed]
35. Babu, K.M.; Haddad, Y.K.; Causey, S.T.; Vargas-Torres, C.C.; Martinez, P.M.; Goldberg, E.M.; Dorfman, J.D.; Bleser, J.A.; Chapman, B.P.; Lai, J.T.; et al. Detection of ethanol, cannabinoids, benzodiazepines, and opioids in older adults evaluated for serious injuries from falls. *Clin. Toxicol.* **2024**, *62*, 661–668. [CrossRef] [PubMed]
36. 2023 American Geriatrics Society Beers Criteria® Update Expert Panel. American Geriatrics Society 2023 updated AGS Beers Criteria® for potentially inappropriate medication use in older adults. *J. Am. Geriatr. Soc.* **2023**, *71*, 2052–2081. [CrossRef] [PubMed]
37. Russell, M.A.; Hill, K.D.; Blackberry, I.; Day, L.L.; Dharmage, S.C. Falls risk and functional decline in older fallers discharged directly from emergency departments. *J. Gerontol. A Biol. Sci. Med. Sci.* **2006**, *61*, 1090–1095. [CrossRef] [PubMed]
38. Carpenter, C.R.; Scheatzle, M.D.; D'Antonio, J.A.; Ricci, P.T.; Coben, J.H. Identification of fall risk factors in older adult emergency department patients. *Acad. Emerg. Med.* **2009**, *16*, 211–219. [CrossRef] [PubMed]
39. Davenport, K.; Alazemi, M.; Sri-On, J.; Liu, S. Missed Opportunities to Diagnose and Intervene in Modifiable Risk Factors for Older Emergency Department Patients Presenting After a Fall. *Ann. Emerg. Med.* **2020**, *76*, 730–738. [CrossRef] [PubMed]
40. Strauss, D.H.; Davoodi, N.M.; Resnik, L.J.; Keene, S.; Serina, P.T.; Goldberg, E.M. Emergency Department-Based Physical Function Measures for Falls in Older Adults and Outcomes: A Secondary Analysis of GAPcare. *J. Geriatr. Phys. Ther.* **2024**, *47*, 137–144. [CrossRef] [PubMed]
41. Hammouda, N.; Carpenter, C.R.; Hung, W.W.; Lesser, A.; Nyamu, S.; Liu, S.; Gettel, C.J.; Malsch, A.; Castillo, E.M.; Forrester, S.; et al. Moving the needle on fall prevention: A Geriatric Emergency Care Applied Research (GEAR) Network scoping review and consensus statement. *Acad. Emerg. Med.* **2021**, *28*, 1214–1227. [CrossRef] [PubMed]
42. Guirguis-Blake, J.M.; Perdue, L.A.; Coppola, E.L.; Bean, S.I. Interventions to Prevent Falls in Older Adults: Updated Evidence Report and Systematic Review for the US Preventive Services Task Force. *JAMA* **2024**, *332*, 58–69. [CrossRef] [PubMed]
43. Graves, J.M.; Whitehill, J.M.; Hagel, B.E.; Rivara, F.P. Making the most of injury surveillance data: Using narrative text to identify exposure information in case-control studies. *Injury* **2015**, *46*, 891–897. [CrossRef] [PubMed]
44. Min, J.; Gurka, K.K.; Kalesan, B.; Bian, J.; Prosperi, M. Injury Burden in the United States: Accurate, Reliable, and Timely Surveillance Using Electronic Health Care Data. *Am. J. Public. Health* **2019**, *109*, 1702–1706. [CrossRef] [PubMed]
45. Tom, A.; Schuluttenhofer, A.; Navarro, S.M.; Junker, M.; Zietlow, J.; Davis, R.; Palmer, A.K.; LeBrasseur, N.K.; Bellolio, F.; Park, M. Increasing Incidence and Hospitalization of Bed-Related Fall Injuries in Older Adults. In Proceedings of the American Geriatric Society 2025 Annual Meeting, Chicago, IL, USA, 8–10 May 2025.

Journal of
Clinical Medicine

Article

Anterior Redisplacement After Intramedullary Nail Fixation for Trochanteric Femoral Fractures: Incidence and Risk Factors in 598 Older Patients

Hironori Kuroda [1,2], Suguru Yokoo [1,*], Yukimasa Okada [1], Junya Kondo [1], Koji Sakagami [1], Takahiko Ichikawa [1], Keiya Yamana [1] and Chuji Terada [1]

1 Department of Orthopaedic Surgery, Fukuyama City Hospital, Hiroshima 721-8511, Japan; hironori-kuroda@nms.ac.jp (H.K.)
2 Shock and Trauma Center, Nippon Medical School, Chiba Hokusoh Hospital, Inzai 270-1694, Japan
* Correspondence: d04sm100@gmail.com; Tel.: +81-84-941-5151; Fax: +81-84-941-5159

Abstract: Background/Objectives: Anterior redisplacement, defined as a postoperative anterior shift of the distal fragment despite intraoperative reduction, is occasionally observed after cephalomedullary nailing for trochanteric femoral fractures. However, its incidence and associated risk factors remain unclear. This study aimed to determine the incidence of anterior redisplacement following intramedullary nail fixation in geriatric trochanteric fractures, and to identify independent risk factors. **Methods:** This study retrospectively reviewed data from 598 consecutive hips in 577 patients (aged ≥65 years) who underwent intramedullary nail fixation for trochanteric fractures at a single center (2012–2023). Sagittal reduction on the lateral radiographic view was classified as posterior, anatomical, or anterior according to the position of the distal fragment, and was recorded preoperatively and postoperatively. Anterior redisplacement, the primary outcome, was defined as a change in alignment from a posterior or anatomical position postoperatively to an anterior position on any subsequent follow-up radiograph. Independent risk factors were identified by logistic regression. **Results:** Among the 543 hips reduced posteriorly ($n = 204$) or anatomically ($n = 339$), anterior redisplacement occurred in 73 (13.4%). The incidence of anterior redisplacement was significantly higher following anatomical compared to posterior reduction (19.5% vs. 3.4%; $p < 0.001$), and also higher in fractures that were anteriorly aligned preoperatively (18.0%) compared to anatomical (8.5%; $p < 0.01$) and posterior (6.2%; $p < 0.01$) alignment. Multivariate analysis revealed two independent predictors: preoperative anterior alignment (odds ratio [OR] 1.87, 95% confidence interval [CI] 1.24–2.81; $p = 0.003$) and postoperative anatomical (vs. posterior) reduction (OR 6.49, 95% CI 2.92–14.44; $p < 0.001$). Age, sex, Arbeitsgemeinschaft für Osteosynthesefragen/Orthopaedic Trauma Association classification, Evans–Jensen classification, nail length, and canal-filling ratio were not associated with redisplacement. No lag-screw cutout occurred during the follow-up. **Conclusions:** Anterior redisplacement occurred in one of seven geriatric trochanteric fractures despite apparently satisfactory fixation. An anatomical sagittal reduction—traditionally considered "ideal"—increases the risk more than sixfold, whereas a deliberate posterior-buttress is protective. Unlike patient-related risk factors, sagittal reduction is under the surgeon's control. The study findings provide evidence that choosing a slight posterior bias can significantly improve stability.

https://doi.org/10.3390/jcm14155557

Keywords: hip fractures; aged; femoral fractures; bone nails; fracture fixation; internal; reoperation; treatment failure; postoperative complications

1. Introduction

Worldwide, intertrochanteric fractures account for roughly half of the 6–7 million hip fractures projected annually by 2050. Most occur in adults aged ≥65 years and are associated with 30-day and 1-year mortality rates of 10% and 20%–30%, respectively [1]. Recent Japanese epidemiological data demonstrate a persistent rise in proximal femoral fractures, with 2005–2014 surveillance documenting a steadily increasing incidence [2]. A 35-year prefectural cohort study further reported 3369 hip fractures in 2020 alongside a pronounced rebound in individuals aged ≥90 years [3]. The resulting loss of independent mobility increases the institutional care demand and generates direct medical costs exceeding USD 20 billion annually in high-income countries [4]. A more recent European report showed that fragility fractures in the EU27+2 region incurred direct healthcare costs of EUR 56.9 billion in 2019—an increase of approximately USD 2000–5000 per case compared with earlier estimates [5].

Failed cephalomedullary fixation—particularly lag-screw or helical-blade cutout—remains the most devastating mechanical complication, requiring revision arthroplasty in up to 7% of cases [6]. In a recent multicenter nested case–control study (n = 2327), Inui et al. reported that anterior malreduction—defined as anterior displacement of the distal fragment on postoperative oblique–lateral radiographs—increased the risk of cutout independently of the tip–apex distance [7]. Although the tip–apex distance is a well-established predictor of cutout, their findings shed new light on the independent effect of anterior malreduction, emphasizing its clinical relevance.

Especially in older adults, closed reduction is generally preferred to minimize surgical invasiveness. Moreover, recent studies suggest that closed reduction may also attenuate postoperative sterile inflammatory responses [8]. However, achieving satisfactory sagittal alignment through closed methods alone can be technically challenging. Numerous intraoperative techniques have been developed to assist sagittal reduction in trochanteric fractures, including reduction tools, percutaneous pins, and clamp-based methods. These approaches are particularly useful when satisfactory alignment cannot be achieved by closed manipulation alone [9–12].

Despite apparently acceptable intraoperative images, clinicians continue to observe anterior redisplacement on early follow-up radiographs [13]. This phenomenon indicates that static malreduction explains only part of the failure mechanism; fracture segments may move secondarily through lag-screw telescoping or posterior sagging before the cortical buttress engages [14,15]. However, the incidence, predictors, and clinical consequences of this dynamic instability have not been quantified in a large cohort.

We hypothesized that fractures initially presenting with an anterior alignment—or reduced to a neutral (anatomical) rather than posterior-buttress position—would exhibit higher rates of anterior redisplacement and, consequently, greater mechanical instability. To test this hypothesis, the position of the bone fragments was evaluated at three distinct time points—preoperatively, immediately postoperatively, and at follow-up—allowing us to identify any anterior redisplacement over time.

2. Materials and Methods

2.1. Ethics

The study was conducted according to the guidelines of the Declaration of Helsinki and approved by the Institutional Review Board of Fukuyama City Hospital (Approval number 846 dated 29 November 2024). The requirement for written informed consent was waived by the IRB; instead, participants or their guardians were informed about the study via an opt-out notice posted on our hospital website and displayed within the hospital. Data were securely stored in an encrypted hospital database, accessible only to authorized researchers.

2.2. Study Design, Setting, and Participants

This single-center, retrospective cohort study included 598 hips from 577 patients aged ≥65 years who underwent intramedullary nail fixation for trochanteric femoral fractures at our institution between January 2012 and December 2023 (Figure 1). The primary objectives were to (i) determine the incidence of anterior redisplacement, (ii) identify preoperative and postoperative risk factors, and (iii) clarify its association with implant failure.

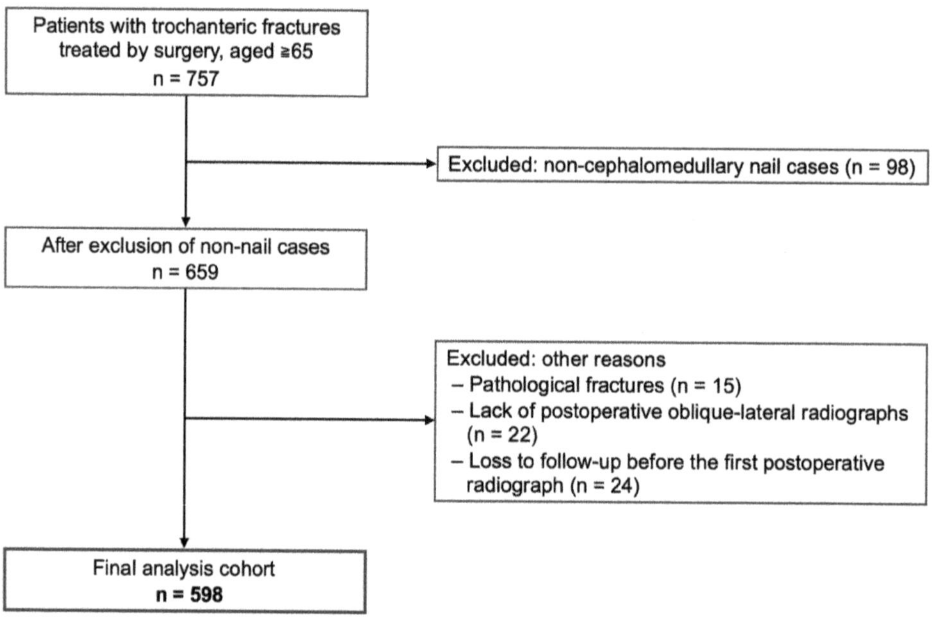

Figure 1. Flow diagram of patient selection.

The exclusion criteria were as follows: (1) pathological fractures, (2) lack of postoperative oblique-lateral radiographs, and (3) loss to follow-up before the first postoperative radiograph was taken. After exclusion, 598 hips of 577 patients constituted the final study cohort. Twenty-one patients sustained metachronous contralateral fractures, i.e., the second hip fracture occurred at a different time and required a separate admission. Each patient contributed two hips, which were analyzed as independent observations because the study focused on hip-specific factors. To analyze anterior redisplacement, we stratified the data by postoperative reduction subtype. As anterior redisplacement was defined as a shift from a posterior or anatomical to an anterior position, hips that were already in an anterior position postoperatively were not eligible for this analysis. In accordance with our institution's protocol, patients were transferred to a rehabilitation facility approximately 2 weeks after surgery, returned for clinical and radiographic assessment at 3 months postoperatively, and were followed-up at 6 and 12 months.

2.3. Surgical Technique

All procedures were performed with the patient in the supine position on a traction table under C-arm fluoroscopic guidance. When closed reduction proved difficult, a small lateral incision was made to allow open the reduction of the fracture fragments. Then, an antegrade cephalomedullary nail was inserted through a small proximal window at the apex of the greater trochanter. Detailed implant information is provided in Supplementary Table S1.

2.4. Radiographic Classification

Standard anteroposterior and oblique-lateral radiographs of the hip were obtained before surgery, immediately after surgery, at 1 week after surgery, and at routine follow-up visits as determined by the treating physician.

Sagittal reduction on the oblique-lateral radiographic view was classified into three subtypes (Figure 2):

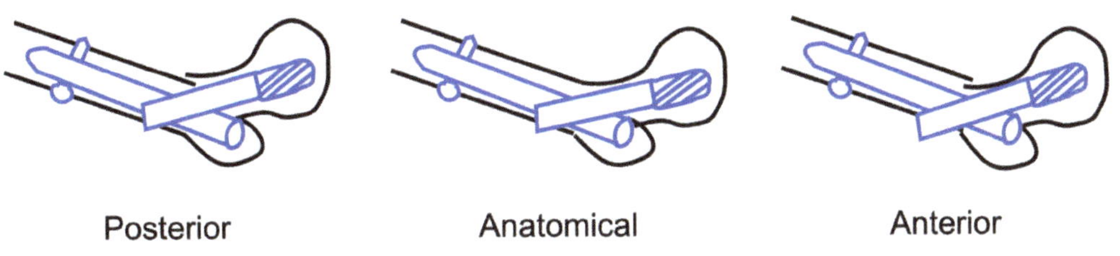

Figure 2. Schematic of the sagittal reduction subtypes on oblique-lateral radiographs.

Posterior—the distal fragment lies posterior to the proximal fragment;

Anatomical—the cortices of the two fragments are co-linear;

Anterior—the anterior cortex of the distal fragment lies anterior to the anterior cortex of the proximal fragment.

2.5. Outcomes

The primary outcome was anterior redisplacement, defined as the postoperative migration of a distal fracture segment that had been reduced in an anatomical or posterior position to an anterior position on any follow-up radiograph. The secondary outcome was lag-screw cutout; however, no cutout events occurred during follow-up. Therefore, this endpoint is described but not formally analyzed.

2.6. Covariates

The following potential confounders were extracted from the medical records and radiographs: age, sex, comorbidities, Arbeitsgemeinschaft für Osteosynthesefragen/Orthopaedic Trauma Association (AO/OTA) classification (31A1/A2/A3) [16], Evans–Jensen classification (I–V) [17], nail length (short, <230 mm; middle, 230–260 mm; and long >260 mm), canal-filling ratio (defined as the ratio of the nail diameter to the canal diameter measured on both anteroposterior and oblique-lateral radiographs—at 1 cm proximal to the nail tip for short nails and at the narrowest point of the canal for middle and long nails), and the preoperative sagittal subtype described above.

2.7. Statistical Analysis

Continuous variables were tested for normality using the Shapiro–Wilk test. Continuous variables are presented as mean ± standard deviation and were compared through Student's t-test or Welch's t-test, depending on the equality of variances. Categorical variables, which were compared by Fisher's exact test, are reported as counts with percentages. Variables associated with anterior redisplacement in the univariate analysis ($p < 0.05$) were simultaneously entered into a multivariate logistic regression model. The results are expressed as odds ratios (ORs) with 95% confidence intervals (CIs). Model calibration was assessed using the Hosmer–Lemeshow goodness-of-fit test. A two-sided p-value < 0.05 was considered significant. All analyses were performed using EZR (Easy R) version 2.73 (Saitama Medical Center, Jichi Medical University, Saitama, Japan), which is a graphical user interface for R (The R Foundation for Statistical Computing, Vienna, Austria).

3. Results

3.1. Patient Demographics

During the study period, a total of 598 hips (mean age, 85.6 ± 7.6 years; 444 women and 154 men) underwent intramedullary nail fixation for trochanteric femoral fractures. Baseline comorbidities included cardiovascular disease in 197 hips, renal disease in 96, pulmonary disease in 65, cerebrovascular disease in 123, and dementia in 151 (Table 1).

Table 1. Baseline characteristics of the study population (n = 598).

Variable	
Number of cases	598
Sex (female/male)	444/154
Age, years (mean ± SD)	85.8 ± 7.5
Comorbidities	
Cardiovascular disease	197
Renal disease	96
Pulmonary disease	65
Cerebrovascular disease	123
Dementia	151
AO/OTA classification	
A1	259
A2	268
A3	71
Evans–Jensen classification	
I	23
II	58
III	217
IV	13
V	287
Nail length	
Short (<230 mm)	435
Middle (230 to <260 mm)	98
Long (>260 mm)	65
Preoperative subtype	
Posterior	109
Anatomical	151
Anterior	338
Filling ratio (mean ± SD)	
Anteroposterior view	0.80 ± 0.10
Oblique-lateral view	0.70 ± 0.10

Abbreviations: SD, standard deviation; AO/OTA, Arbeitsgemeinschaft für Osteosynthesefragen/Orthopaedic Trauma Association.

Various cephalomedullary nails were used, such as InterTAN® ($n = 302$; Smith & Nephew, Memphis, TN, USA), IPT® ($n = 112$; HOMS, Tokyo, Japan), PFNA® ($n = 109$; DePuy Synthes, Zuchwil, Switzerland), and others. Details of all implant types and manufacturers are provided in Table S1.

The subtypes of the preoperative sagittal alignment were posterior in 109 hips (18.2%), anatomical in 151 (25.2%), and anterior in 338 (56.5%).

3.2. Incidence of Anterior Redisplacement

Among all 598 fractures, 204 (34.1%), 339 (56.7%), and 55 (9.1%) were reduced to posterior, anatomical, and anterior positions, respectively, on the postoperative radiograph. Given that fractures that had already reduced anteriorly could not translate further anteriorly, these 55 hips were excluded, leaving 543 evaluable hips for the redisplacement analysis.

Among the 543 hips analyzed, posterior reduction was achieved significantly more often in female patients, in fractures classified as more complex by the AO and Evans–Jensen systems, and in cases treated with middle or long intramedullary nails (Table 2).

Table 2. Characteristics of patients showing posterior or anatomical reductions in postoperative radiograph.

Variable	All ($n = 543$)	Posterior ($n = 204$)	Anatomical ($n = 339$)	p-Value
Sex				0.02
Female	411	166	245	
Male	132	38	94	
Age, years (mean ± SD)	85.8 ± 7.6	86.2 ± 7.6	85.5 ± 7.6	0.29
Comorbidities				
Cardiovascular disease	181	69	112	0.85
Renal disease	85	33	52	0.81
Pulmonary disease	62	25	37	0.68
Cerebrovascular disease	113	45	68	0.59
Dementia	141	49	92	0.48
AO/OTA classification				0.02
A1	231	71	160	
A2	249	105	144	
A3	63	28	35	
Evans–Jensen classification				0.001
I	23	2	21	
II	54	14	40	
III	185	65	120	
IV	12	5	7	
V	269	118	151	
Nail length				0.001
Short (<230 mm)	390	130	260	
Middle (230 to <260 mm)	93	50	43	
Long (>260 mm)	60	24	36	
Filling ratio (mean ± SD)				
Anteroposterior view	0.80 ± 0.10	0.80 ± 0.10	0.81 ± 0.10	0.46
Oblique-lateral view	0.70 ± 0.10	0.71 ± 0.10	0.70 ± 0.10	0.09

Abbreviations: SD, standard deviation; AO/OTA, Arbeitsgemeinschaft für Osteosynthesefragen/Orthopaedic Trauma Association. Patient characteristics stratified by postoperative sagittal reduction. Posterior reduction was more commonly observed in female patients, who are presumed to have more osteoporotic bone, and in those with more complex fracture types based on the AO/OTA and Evans–Jensen classifications. Additionally, longer nails (middle or long) were more frequently used in the posterior group, which may reflect the surgeon's intraoperative assessment of greater mechanical instability.

Overall, anterior redisplacement occurred in 73 of 543 (13.4%) hips. No significant associations were found between anterior redisplacement and age, sex, AO/OTA, Evans–Jensen classification, nail length, or filling ratio (all $p > 0.05$; Table 3).

Table 3. Characteristics of patients with anterior redisplacement after surgery.

Variable	All (n = 543)	Anterior Redisplacement (n = 73)	No Redisplacement (n = 470)	p-Value
Sex				0.77
Female	411	54	357	
Male	132	19	113	
Age, years (mean ± SD)	85.8 ± 7.6	85.4 ± 7.6	85.8 ± 7.6	0.68
Comorbidities				
Cardiovascular disease	181	19	162	0.18
Renal disease	85	13	72	0.60
Pulmonary disease	62	8	54	1.0
Cerebrovascular disease	113	16	97	0.76
Dementia	141	17	124	0.67
AO/OTA classification				1.00
A1	231	31	200	
A2	249	34	215	
A3	63	8	55	
Evans–Jensen classification				0.26
I	23	1	22	
II	54	5	49	
III	185	22	163	
IV	12	3	9	
V	269	42	227	
Evans–Jensen classification				0.12
I + II	77	6	71	
III − V	469	67	399	
Nail length				0.74
Short (<230 mm)	390	55	335	
Middle (230 to < 260 mm)	93	10	83	
Long (>260 mm)	60	8	52	
Filling ratio (mean ± SD)				
Anteroposterior view	0.80 ± 0.10	0.80 ± 0.10	0.81 ± 0.09	0.67
Oblique-lateral view	0.70 ± 0.10	0.70 ± 0.10	0.69 ± 0.09	0.39

Abbreviations: SD, standard deviation; AO/OTA, Arbeitsgemeinschaft für Osteosynthesefragen/Orthopaedic Trauma Association. No significant associations were observed for age, comorbidities, fracture classification, or implant characteristics (all $p > 0.05$).

Preoperative sagittal alignment influenced the risk of redisplacement (Figure 3, Table 4). The incidence rates were 6.2% (6/97), 8.5% (12/141), and 18.0% (55/305) in patients with preoperative posterior, anatomical, and anterior subtypes, respectively (overall, p = 0.0016; pairwise $p < 0.01$ for posterior vs. anterior and anatomical vs. anterior).

Table 4. Incidence of anterior redisplacement according to the preoperative alignment subtype.

Preoperative Subtype	Anterior Translation (+)	Anterior Translation (−)	Total	Incidence (%)	p-Value
Posterior	6	91	97	6.2%	-
Anatomical	12	129	141	8.5%	-
Anterior	55	250	305	18.0%	0.0016
Total	73	470	543	13.4%	

The incidence of anterior redisplacement varied significantly by preoperative sagittal alignment, occurring in 6.2%, 8.5%, and 18.0% of hips with posterior, anatomical, and anterior subtypes, respectively (overall p = 0.0005; pairwise $p < 0.01$ for posterior vs. anterior and anatomical vs. anterior).

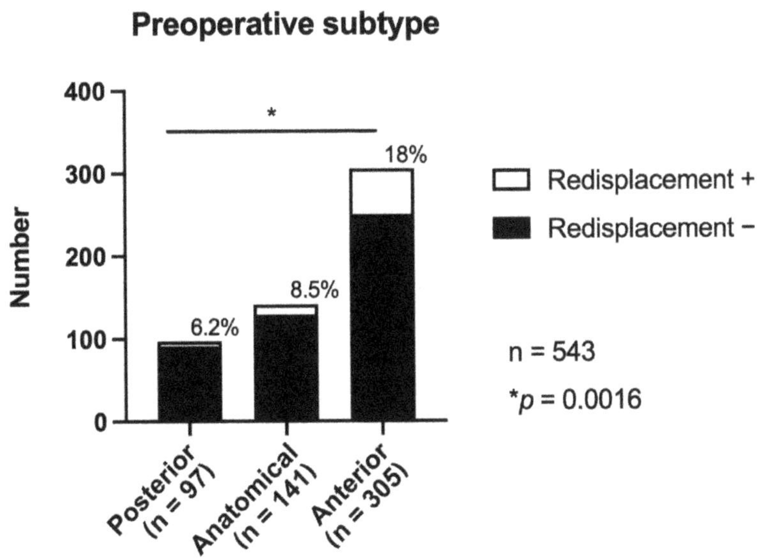

Figure 3. Incidence of anterior redisplacement according to the preoperative alignment subtype.

Postoperative sagittal reduction showed a strong association with anterior redisplacement (Figure 4, Table 5). Anterior redisplacement was significantly more frequent in anatomical reduction than in posteriorly reduced hips (19.5% [66/339] vs. 3.4% [7/204]; $p < 0.0001$).

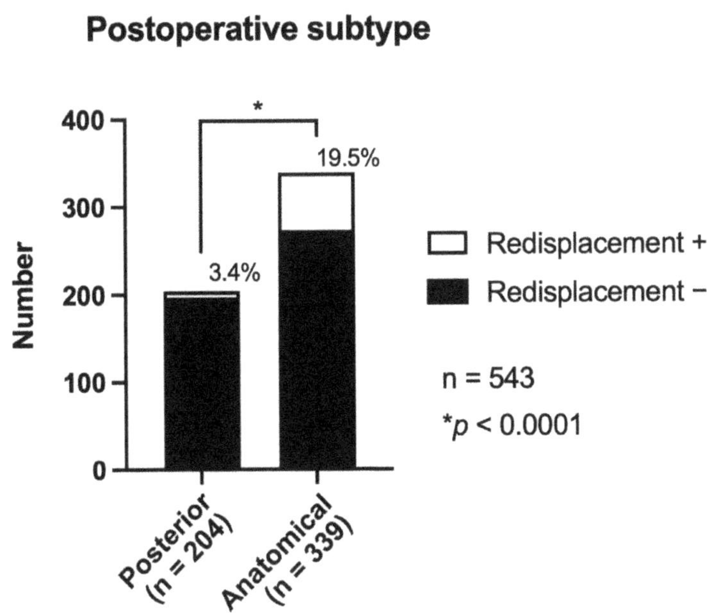

Figure 4. Incidence of anterior redisplacement according to the postoperative reduction subtype.

Table 5. Incidence of anterior redisplacement according to the postoperative reduction subtype.

Preoperative Subtype	Anterior Translation (+)	Anterior Translation (−)	Total	Incidence (%)	*p*-Value
Posterior	7	197	204	3.4%	<0.0001
Anatomical	66	273	339	19.5%	-
Total	73	470	543	13.4%	

The white portions of the bars represent cases with anterior redisplacement, whereas the black portions represent cases without redisplacement. The percentage above each bar indicates the incidence of redisplacement in that group—6.2%, 8.5%, and 18.0% in the posteriorly, anatomically, and anteriorly aligned groups, respectively. The overall comparison across subtypes was significant (* $p = 0.0016$, Fisher's exact test). The total number of cases $n = 543$.

Incidence of anterior redisplacement according to the postoperative reduction subtype. The anatomically reduced group exhibited a significantly higher incidence of redisplacement (19.5%) than the posteriorly reduced group (3.4%) ($p < 0.0001$).

The incidence was significantly higher in the anatomically reduced group (19.5%) than in the posteriorly reduced group (3.4%). Cases with the postoperative anterior subtype ($n = 55$) were excluded from this analysis.

3.3. Multivariate Analysis

Multivariate logistic regression identified two independent risk factors for anterior redisplacement (Table 6), namely, preoperative anterior position (vs. non-anterior) with an OR of 1.87 (95% CI: 1.24–2.81, $p = 0.003$) and postoperative anatomical reduction (vs. posterior) with an OR 6.49 (95% CI: 2.92–14.44, $p < 0.001$). The model showed acceptable calibration (Hosmer–Lemeshow, $\chi^2 = 7.265$, $p = 0.123$), with a Nagelkerke R^2 of 0.134, and correctly classified 86.5% of the cases.

Table 6. Multivariate logistic regression analysis of the risk factors for anterior redisplacement.

Variable	OR (95% CI)	*p*-Value
Preoperative anterior position (vs. non-anterior)	1.87 (1.24–2.81)	0.003
Postoperative anatomical reduction (vs. posterior)	6.49 (2.92–14.44)	<0.0001

Abbreviations: OR, odds ratio; CI, confidence interval.

These results indicate that an anteriorly displaced fracture pattern before surgery and an anatomical (rather than posterior) sagittal reduction following intramedullary nailing markedly increase the risk of anterior redisplacement during follow-up.

Reference categories: preoperative position = non-anterior (anatomical/posterior); postoperative reduction = posterior reduction.

In the multivariate logistic regression (Table 6), both preoperative anterior position and postoperative anatomical reduction were independent predictors of anterior redisplacement. Specifically, a preoperative anterior position was associated with a 1.87-fold increase in the odds of redisplacement (OR 1.87, 95% CI 1.24–2.81; $p = 0.003$), and anatomical postoperative reduction conferred a 6.49-fold higher OR than posterior reduction (OR 6.49, 95% CI 2.92–14.44; $p < 0.001$).

4. Discussion

4.1. Principal Findings

In this large, single-center cohort of 598 hips from older patients who underwent intramedullary nailing for the treatment of trochanteric femoral fractures, anterior redisplacement occurred in 13.4% of the 543 hips that had been reduced in either an anatomical or the posterior position. Multivariate analysis identified two independent and clinically actionable risk factors—a preoperative anterior fracture alignment almost doubled the odds of redisplacement (OR: 1.87), and a postoperative anatomical reduction increased the odds more than sixfold compared with posterior reduction (OR: 6.49) (Table 6). Neither fracture morphology (AO/OTA and Evans–Jensen classification) nor implant-related variables (nail length and filling ratio) were associated with redisplacement (Table 3). Taken together, these findings indicate that sagittal alignment—particularly the surgeon-controlled achievement of a slight posterior reduction—outweighs implant choice and fracture complexity as the dominant, modifiable determinant of postoperative stability.

Compared with hips reduced to an anatomical position, posterior reduction on postoperative radiographs was more frequently observed in female patients, in those with more complex fracture patterns, and in those treated using middle or long nails (Table 2). These patterns largely reflect the surgeon's preference; posterior alignment was deliberately selected for female patients with osteoporosis and those with unstable fractures. This selection bias may have influenced the final outcomes because posterior reduction was more likely achieved in cases where postoperative redisplacement was already of concern.

4.2. Pathophysiological Interpretation

Postoperative anterior redisplacement occurs when the distal shaft fragment does not lie posterior to the head–neck fragment, leaving the anteromedial cortex unsupported. Under axial loading, this produces a sagittal-swing moment that drives the proximal fragment further into flexion. Once the lag-screw telescopes, secondary sliding amplifies the displacement and shortens the neck [13,18,19]. In contrast, placing the head–neck fragment slightly posterior ($\leq$1 cortical thickness) to the shaft establishes an anteromedial buttress that converts shear into compression and allows the sharing of loads between the bone and the nail. Biomechanical tests have shown that compared with an intramedullary (anterior) reduction, this "extramedullary" or "positive medial cortical support" configuration halves telescoping and reduces nail migration [20,21]. In the present cohort, such posterior over-reduction lowered the odds of redisplacement sixfold (OR: 6.49).

To our knowledge, this study is the first to investigate the relationship between preoperative displacement and the postoperative loss of reduction. Patients presenting with anterior shift of the distal segment preoperatively were more likely to experience postoperative redisplacement, even when anatomical or posterior reduction was achieved (Tables 4 and S2). This finding may suggest an inherent instability in fracture patterns that initially present with anterior displacement.

4.3. Comparison with Previous Studies

Most studies have focused on coronal alignment and the tip–apex distance, with relatively few large-scale analyses of sagittal reduction and postoperative redisplacement [7,22]. Biomechanical and small clinical reports have shown that anterior malreduction increases the risk of lag-screw cutout and implant sliding, whereas positive medial cortical support limits impaction and pain [13,19,20]. Although no cutout events occurred in the study cohort and functional outcomes were not assessed systematically, these data collectively suggest that avoiding anterior redisplacement remains a prudent surgical objective.

More recent series have identified dynamic risk factors for redisplacement—comminution at the greater trochanter and low lateral canal-filling ratio [23]; however, in our cohort, the filling ratio was not predictive, and Evans–Jensen type III–V fractures did not exhibit greater instability (Table 3). This highlights the primacy of anteromedial buttress over fracture morphology. However, posterior reduction was more often applied in cases with presumed greater instability, which may have influenced these results (Table 2).

Several recent studies have employed three-dimensional computed tomography to characterize sagittal fragment alignment and cortical buttress formation more precisely [14,23,24], an approach not employed in the present radiograph-based analysis.

By modeling both preoperative and postoperative sagittal alignment within a single logistic framework in the largest uniform radiograph-based cohort to date (n = 598), this study clarified their independent and additive contributions to postoperative stability. This study extends this literature in three ways, by (i) evaluating dynamic redisplacement rather than static malreduction, capturing fractures that were acceptable intraoperatively but destabilized during early loading; (ii) modeling preoperative and postoperative alignment within the same logistic framework, clarifying their independent and additive contributions to instability; and (iii) analyzing the largest single-institution cohort to date (n = 598) with uniform imaging and follow-up, thereby narrowing the CIs around the effect estimates. Importantly, the fact that Evans–Jensen type III–V fractures did not exhibit higher redisplacement rates (Table 3) underscores the critical importance of support at the thick anteromedial cortex, irrespective of posterior comminution.

4.4. Clinical Implications: Why a Deliberate Posterior Reduction Deserves Routine Consideration

The present findings, together with converging biomechanical and clinical evidence [7,18,19,25], challenge the traditional goal of an anatomically flush sagittal cortex and support a controlled posterior offset, defined as leaving the head–neck fragment ≤1 cortical thickness posterior to the shaft. Leaving the head–neck fragment slightly posterior to the shaft (i) transforms shear into compressive loading across the buttress, (ii) limits telescoping to <2 mm, thus preventing the 5–10 mm of uncontrolled shortening often seen after "anatomical" reductions, and (iii) mitigates varus drift and lag-screw cutout risk. Importantly, this target position is easy to visualize intraoperatively; a 30° oblique-lateral radiographic view should show the distal anteromedial cortex overlapping the proximal spike [26]. When closed manipulation yields a flush or anterior cortex, surgeons should favor a deliberate posterior over-reduction—achievable with a small anteriorly directed elevator—rather than additional traction or nail exchange. Incorporating an item such as "anteromedial cortical buttress achieved (yes/no)" into intraoperative checklists, alongside the tip–apex distance and neck–shaft angle, may facilitate the consistent adoption of this technique.

Although implant failure was rare in our cohort, anterior redisplacement has been linked in previous studies to increased hip pain, delayed weight-bearing, and a higher risk of lag-screw cut-out [7,14,19]. Because posterior reduction is a simple, low-cost maneuver that can be adopted intraoperatively, minimizing redisplacement may still yield meaningful patient benefits even when catastrophic failures are uncommon.

4.5. Strengths and Limitations

The strengths are related to the study being the largest single-center series to date, the use of uniform surgical techniques, blinded radiographic adjudication, and multivariable modeling that separates preoperative and postoperative alignment.

Limitations are intrinsic to the study design, and include the following:

1. Single-institution, retrospective cohort—practice patterns may differ elsewhere; selection and information bias cannot be fully excluded;
2. Follow-up heterogeneity—although 92% of patients had $\geq$3 months of imaging data, late attrition may underestimate very delayed redisplacement;
3. Unmeasured confounders—bone density, surgeon experience, and rehabilitation protocols were not captured; each could influence stability.
   These caveats tamper the generalizability of our numeric risk estimates, but not the biomechanical principle that the anteromedial buttress matters;
4. Clinical outcomes—functional or symptomatic endpoints—including walking capacity, pain, and quality-of-life scores—were not systematically captured in this retrospective cohort. Although lag-screw cut-out was predefined as a secondary endpoint, no such failures were observed, and postoperative lag-screw telescoping was not quantified. Prospective studies that collect patient-reported outcome measures and correlate them with the degree of anterior redisplacement are therefore warranted.

4.6. Future Directions

Prospective, multicenter trials should examine deliberate posterior-biased reduction versus anatomical reduction with standardized implants, rehabilitation, and longer (>12 months) follow-up. Embedding intraoperative motion analysis—for example, optical tracking of fragment drift between reduction and wound closure—could identify micro-instability invisible on two-dimensional fluoroscopy. Finally, finite-element and cadaver models integrating patient-specific bone density may clarify how much posterior offset is optimal for different fracture patterns.

5. Conclusions

Preoperative anterior fracture alignment and postoperative anatomical reduction are independent, clinically significant risk factors for anterior redisplacement following intramedullary nailing of trochanteric femoral fractures in older patients. Achieving—or deliberately leaving—a slight posterior reduction offers a simple, readily modifiable strategy to mitigate this complication, and may translate into better functional outcomes and fewer implant failures.

Supplementary Materials: The following supporting information can be downloaded at: https://www.mdpi.com/article/10.3390/jcm14155557/s1, Table S1. Cephalomedullary nail implants used in the study population: device names, manufacturers, and number of cases. Table S2. Preoperative and postoperative subtypes with the number and percentage of anterior redisplacement cases.

Author Contributions: Conceptualization, H.K., S.Y. and C.T.; methodology, H.K., S.Y. and C.T.; software, H.K. and S.Y.; validation, H.K.; formal analysis, H.K. and S.Y.; investigation, H.K.; data curation, H.K. and S.Y.; writing—original draft preparation, H.K. and S.Y.; writing—review and editing, H.K., S.Y., Y.O., J.K., K.S., T.I., K.Y. and C.T.; visualization, H.K. and S.Y.; supervision, S.Y., Y.O., K.Y. and C.T.; project administration, C.T. All authors have read and agreed to the published version of the manuscript.

Funding: This research received no external funding.

Institutional Review Board Statement: The study was conducted according to the guidelines of the Declaration of Helsinki and approved by the Institutional Review Board of Fukuyama City Hospital (Approval number 846 dated 29 November 2024).

Informed Consent Statement: Patient consent was waived due to the requirement for written informed consent being waived by the IRB.

Data Availability Statement: Due to ethical considerations, we are unable to make the full dataset publicly available. However, we are open to discussing requests for anonymized data from qualified researchers under appropriate agreements.

Acknowledgments: The authors would like to acknowledge our institution for their contributions to the study, including support with patient data collection and surgical expertise. All authors have read and agreed to the published version of the manuscript.

Conflicts of Interest: The authors declare no conflicts of interest.

References

1. Dong, Y.; Zhang, Y.; Song, K.; Kang, H.; Ye, D.; Li, F. What was the Epidemiology and Global Burden of Disease of Hip Fractures from 1990 to 2019? Results from and Additional Analysis of the Global Burden of Disease Study 2019. *Clin. Orthop. Relat. Res.* **2023**, *481*, 1209–1220. [CrossRef]
2. Shoji, A.; Gao, Z.; Arai, K.; Yoshimura, N. 30-year trends of hip and vertebral fracture incidence in Japan: A systematic review and meta-analysis. *J. Bone Miner. Metab.* **2022**, *40*, 327–336. [CrossRef] [PubMed]
3. Nozaki, A.; Imai, N.; Shobugawa, Y.; Suzuki, H.; Horigome, Y.; Endo, N.; Kawashima, H. Increased incidence among the very elderly in the 2020 Niigata Prefecture Osteoporotic Hip Fracture Study. *J. Bone Miner. Metab.* **2023**, *41*, 533–541. [CrossRef] [PubMed]
4. Hernlund, E.; Svedbom, A.; Ivergard, M.; Compston, J.; Cooper, C.; Stenmark, J.; McCloskey, E.V.; Jonsson, B.; Kanis, J.A. Osteoporosis in the European Union: Medical management, epidemiology and economic burden. A report prepared in collaboration with the International Osteoporosis Foundation (IOF) and the European Federation of Pharmaceutical Industry Associations (EFPIA). *Arch. Osteoporos.* **2013**, *8*, 136. [CrossRef] [PubMed]
5. Kanis, J.A.; Norton, N.; Harvey, N.C.; Jacobson, T.; Johansson, H.; Lorentzon, M.; McCloskey, E.V.; Willers, C.; Borgstrom, F. SCOPE 2021: A new scorecard for osteoporosis in Europe. *Arch. Osteoporos.* **2021**, *16*, 82. [CrossRef]
6. Li, S.; Chang, S.M.; Niu, W.X.; Ma, H. Comparison of tip apex distance and cut-out complications between helical blades and lag screws in intertrochanteric fractures among the elderly: A meta-analysis. *J. Orthop. Sci.* **2015**, *20*, 1062–1069.
7. Inui, T.; Watanabe, Y.; Suzuki, T.; Matsui, K.; Kurata, Y.; Ishii, K.; Kurozumi, T.; Kawano, H. Anterior Malreduction is Associated with Lag Screw Cutout After Internal Fixation of Intertrochanteric Fractures. *Clin. Orthop. Relat. Res.* **2024**, *482*, 536–545. [CrossRef]
8. Moldovan, F. Sterile Inflammatory Response and Surgery-Related Trauma in Elderly Patients with Subtrochanteric Fractures. *Biomedicines* **2024**, *12*, 354. [CrossRef]
9. Chun, Y.S.; Oh, H.; Cho, Y.J.; Rhyu, K.H. Technique and early results of percutaneous reduction of sagittally unstable intertrochateric fractures. *Clin. Orthop. Surg.* **2011**, *3*, 217–224. [CrossRef]
10. Kim, Y.; Dheep, K.; Lee, J.; Yoon, Y.C.; Shon, W.Y.; Oh, C.W.; Oh, J.K. Hook leverage technique for reduction of intertrochanteric fracture. *Injury* **2014**, *45*, 1006–1010. [CrossRef]
11. Qiu, J.; Jiang, Z.; Han, L.; Li, X.; Zhang, R.; Wu, B.; Zhu, F.; Zhao, Y. Treatment of irreducible intertrochanteric femoral fracture with a minimally invasive clamp reduction technique via the anterior approach. *J. Orthop. Surg. Res.* **2023**, *18*, 167. [CrossRef]
12. Takigawa, N.; Moriuchi, H.; Abe, M.; Yasui, K.; Eshiro, H.; Kinoshita, M. Complications and fixation techniques of trochanteric fractures with the TARGON((R)) PF. *Injury* **2014**, *45* (Suppl. 1), S44–S48. [CrossRef]
13. Tsukada, S.; Okumura, G.; Matsueda, M. Postoperative stability on lateral radiographs in the surgical treatment of pertrochanteric hip fractures. *Arch. Orthop. Trauma Surg.* **2012**, *132*, 839–846. [CrossRef]
14. Chang, S.M.; Zhang, Y.Q.; Du, S.C.; Ma, Z.; Hu, S.J.; Yao, X.Z.; Xiong, W.F. Anteromedial cortical support reduction in unstable pertrochanteric fractures: A comparison of intra-operative fluoroscopy and post-operative three dimensional computerised tomography reconstruction. *Int. Orthop.* **2018**, *42*, 183–189. [CrossRef]
15. Kim, K.H.; Kang, M.S.; Lim, E.J.; Park, M.L.; Kim, J.J. Posterior Sagging After Cephalomedullary Nailing for Intertrochanteric Femur Fracture is Associated with a Separation of the Greater Trochanter. *Geriatr. Orthop. Surg. Rehabil.* **2020**, *11*, 2151459320946013. [CrossRef] [PubMed]
16. Meinberg, E.G.; Agel, J.; Roberts, C.S.; Karam, M.D.; Kellam, J.F. Fracture and Dislocation Classification Compendium—2018. *J. Orthop. Trauma* **2018**, *32* (Suppl. 1), S1–S170. [CrossRef] [PubMed]
17. Jensen, J.S. Classification of trochanteric fractures. *Acta Orthop. Scand.* **1980**, *51*, 803–810. [CrossRef]
18. Kozono, N.; Ikemura, S.; Yamashita, A.; Harada, T.; Watanabe, T.; Shirasawa, K. Direct reduction may need to be considered to avoid postoperative subtype P in patients with an unstable trochanteric fracture: A retrospective study using a multivariate analysis. *Arch. Orthop. Trauma Surg.* **2014**, *134*, 1649–1654. [CrossRef] [PubMed]

19. Momii, K.; Fujiwara, T.; Mae, T.; Tokunaga, M.; Iwasaki, T.; Shiomoto, K.; Kubota, K.; Onizuka, T.; Miura, T.; Hamada, T.; et al. Risk factors for excessive postoperative sliding of femoral trochanteric fracture in elderly patients: A retrospective multicenter study. *Injury* **2021**, *52*, 3369–3376. [CrossRef]
20. Chang, S.M.; Zhang, Y.Q.; Ma, Z.; Li, Q.; Dargel, J.; Eysel, P. Fracture reduction with positive medial cortical support: A key element in stability reconstruction for the unstable pertrochanteric hip fractures. *Arch. Orthop. Trauma Surg.* **2015**, *135*, 811–818. [CrossRef]
21. Kawamura, T.; Minehara, H.; Tazawa, R.; Matsuura, T.; Sakai, R.; Takaso, M. Biomechanical Evaluation of Extramedullary Versus Intramedullary Reduction in Unstable Femoral Trochanteric Fractures. *Geriatr. Orthop. Surg. Rehabil.* **2021**, *12*, 2151459321998611. [CrossRef] [PubMed]
22. Murena, L.; Moretti, A.; Meo, F.; Saggioro, E.; Barbati, G.; Ratti, C.; Canton, G. Predictors of cut-out after cephalomedullary nail fixation of pertrochanteric fractures: A retrospective study of 813 patients. *Arch. Orthop. Trauma Surg.* **2018**, *138*, 351–359. [CrossRef]
23. Furui, A.; Terada, N.; Mito, K. Mechanical simulation study of postoperative displacement of trochanteric fractures using the finite element method. *J. Orthop. Surg. Res.* **2018**, *13*, 300. [CrossRef]
24. Song, H.; Chang, S.M.; Hu, S.J.; Du, S.C. Low filling ratio of the distal nail segment to the medullary canal is a risk factor for loss of anteromedial cortical support: A case control study. *J. Orthop. Surg. Res.* **2022**, *17*, 27. [CrossRef]
25. Yamamoto, N.; Tsujimoto, Y.; Yokoo, S.; Demiya, K.; Inoue, M.; Noda, T.; Ozaki, T.; Yorifuji, T. Association between Immediate Postoperative Radiographic Findings and Failed Internal Fixation for Trochanteric Fractures: Systematic Review and Meta-Analysis. *J. Clin. Med.* **2022**, *11*, 4879. [CrossRef] [PubMed]
26. Chen, S.Y.; Chang, S.M.; Tuladhar, R.; Wei, Z.; Xiong, W.F.; Hu, S.J.; Du, S.C. A new fluoroscopic view for evaluation of anteromedial cortex reduction quality during cephalomedullary nailing for intertrochanteric femur fractures: The 30 degrees oblique tangential projection. *BMC Musculoskelet. Disord.* **2020**, *21*, 719. [CrossRef] [PubMed]

MDPI AG
Grosspeteranlage 5
4052 Basel
Switzerland
Tel.: +41 61 683 77 34

Journal of Clinical Medicine Editorial Office
E-mail: jcm@mdpi.com
www.mdpi.com/journal/jcm

www.ingramcontent.com/pod-product-compliance
Lightning Source LLC
Chambersburg PA
CBHW062059220926
51850CB00010B/2817
* 9 7 8 3 7 2 5 8 5 4 5 1 6 *